Families on the Go

Families on the Go

Suzie Roberts

Bonneville Books
Springville, Utah

ISBN 13: 978-1-59955-426-6

Published by Bonneville Books, an imprint of Cedar Fort, Inc., 2373 W. 700 S., Springville, UT, 84663
Distributed by Cedar Fort, Inc., www.cedarfort.com

LIBRARY OF CONGRESS CATALOGING-IN-PUBLICATION DATA

Library of Congress Cataloging-in-Publication Data

Roberts, Suzie, 1975-
 Families on the go / Suzie Roberts.
   p. cm.
 Includes index.
 ISBN 978-1-59955-426-6
 1. Dinners and dining. 2. Make-ahead cookery. I. Title.

 TX652.R6356 2010
 641.5'55--dc22

 2010019099

Cover and page design by Angela Olsen
Edited by Melissa J. Caldwell
Cover design © 2011 by Lyle Mortimer

Printed in China

10 9 8 7 6 5 4 3 2 1

Printed on acid-free paper

Our dinner table drama
Is usually the same.
The setting of the table
Isn't a favorite game.
The fighting for the chairs
Or the coveted blue cup
Makes me wonder why
I don't try to tie them up.
"Yuck, I have to eat this?"
Not quite music to my ears—
I should turn the TV on,
And pretend I cannot hear.
We are together briefly;
Our daily tasks provide
Only minutes in a day
To hear each other's highs!
So, I'll not tie them up;
Together we will eat,
Enjoy the time we have,
And consider it a treat!

Acknowledgments

Thanks to my fabulous hubby for always humoring me in my endeavors.

Thanks to my kids for being great and giving me a reason to be creative in trying to simplify our crazy life.

Thanks to my parents for instilling in me the importance of family dinnertime.

Thanks to my friend Nancy for the support and encouragement that I always need to make things like this happen. Also, a million thanks for the editing help.

Thanks to my Make-Ahead Meal group for being the best and sharing my passion for simplifying dinnertime.

Table of Contents

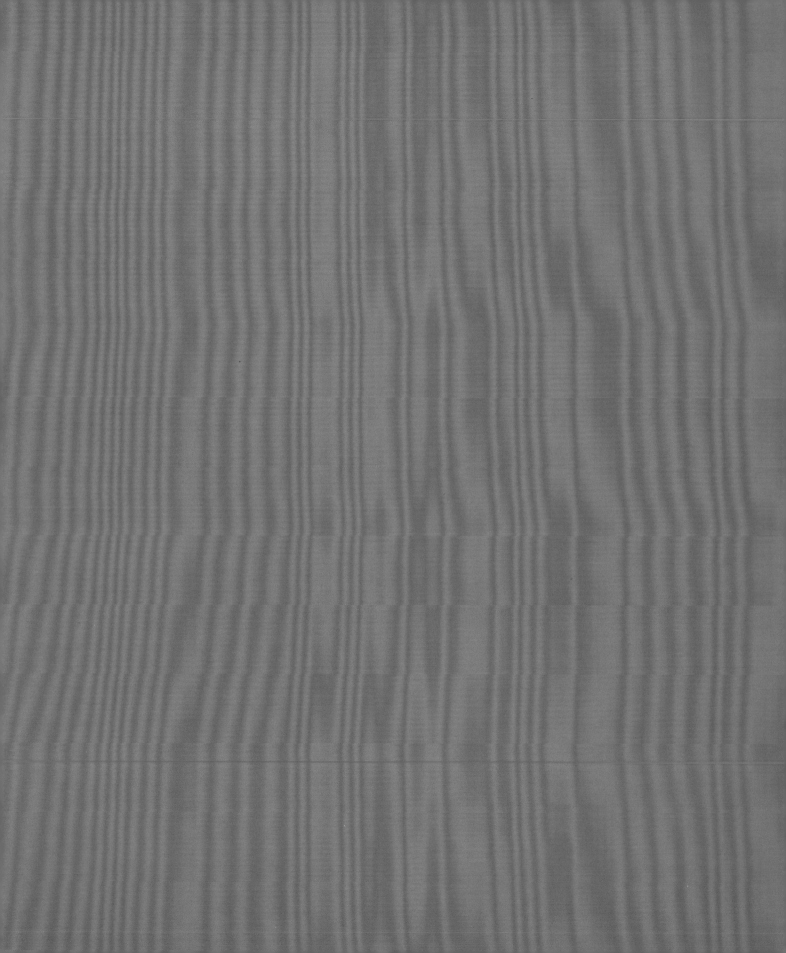

Introduction

Do you sometimes feel like your home is a rest stop? You stop in to have a quick bite to eat, use the restroom, drop off and pick up, and if you're lucky, sometimes you'll run into other family members doing the same thing.

These days, families really have to work to spend time together, so it's important to make every moment together count. This book is for these moments—why to make these moments, ways to make these moments happen, and what to do with these moments when they do happen.

This book is for the family who wants to make memories and traditions, for the family who wants to be stronger and keep memories alive, and for the busy family who wants to enjoy their time together.

Whether you're just looking for some great new meals, trying to simplify, or helping your children remember those great moments, this book helps you achieve your goal. It gives ideas to get the ball rolling to create your own recipe stories and to allow time to make those special memories. It contains many tried-and-true Make-Ahead Meal recipes to give you more time to make memories and enjoy your family.

Good luck in making memories, and always remember—families who eat together keep forever!

The Importance of Eating Together as a Family

Your home is the hub for every family member. The problem is that many times that's all it is. With the craziness of life, there's not much time to eat dinner—let alone eat it together. This chapter will provide some ideas to help you make real, memory-making dinners a reality.

Studies show that parents and children spend only 35.8 minutes a week in meaningful conversation.[1] How do you change that? Family dinner is one way to provide a daily opportunity for meaningful conversation. Although it seems like such a simple thing to eat dinner together as a family, it's easier said than done. Planning and prioritizing play an important part in this attainable goal. Studies have shown that children who do not eat dinner with their families are 61 percent more likely to use alcohol, tobacco, or illegal drugs. By contrast, children who eat dinner with their families every night of the week are 20 percent less likely to drink, smoke, or use illegal drugs.[2] Teens who eat frequent family dinners are less likely than other teens to have sex at young ages, get into fights, or be suspended from school, and they are less likely to contemplate suicide.[3] These studies, among many others available, are overwhelmingly alarming and serve as a reminder that family dinner should be a top priority in the home. But the question remains: how do you accomplish this?

By planning ahead, implementing your family's suggestions, laughing together, and making and recording your dinner memories, you can succeed in making dinnertime a meaningful and wonderful daily family event.

Notes

1. A. C. Nielsen Co., as quoted by "The Importance of Family Dinner," Menu Planning Central, http://www.menuplanningcentral.com/articles/family-dinner.html.
2. Columbia News, "CASA 2000 teen survey: Teens With 'Hands-off' Parents at Four Times Greater Risk of Smoking, Drinking and Using Illegal Drugs as Teens With 'Hands-On' Parents," http://www.columbia.edu/cu/news/01/02/CASA_survey.html.
3. CASA, "Why Family Day?" as found at Family Guide website, "Get Involved: The Importance of Family Mealtime," http://family.samhsa.gov/get/mealtime.aspx?printid=1&.

Family Dinner Ideas

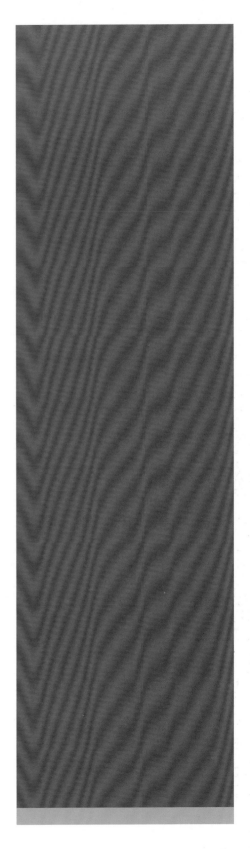

Plan Ahead

First and most important, you must plan ahead. As the saying goes, "If you fail to plan, you plan to fail." And if you do not plan your meals ahead, you will not make eating together a reality.

There are many ways to plan family meals ahead of time; you just need to try out a few until you find what works best for your family. Here are a few ideas:

Make a weekly menu. At the beginning of each week, make a list of the meals you will have each night and the ingredients you need for each of those meals. Then do your grocery shopping for the whole week to cut down on those last-minute grocery store trips.

Make a monthly menu. There are two ways to do this. At the beginning of each month, decide what meals you will make for each day of the month and write it down on your family calendar. This will help you keep it in mind and prepare for it, and it also lets the family know what's for dinner. Another method is to make a list of 25–30 meals and do all your major grocery shopping for the month, so you have the ingredients for all of these meals on the day you need them. Each night, look at your list and decide what you have time to make the next day—or what you're in the mood for! When your calendar for the following day is packed, you can choose something simple off your list. You already have all the ingredients for the meals on your list, so you can choose a meal that you can simply throw in the slow cooker in the morning or assemble just before dinnertime.

Designate a type of meal for each night. Sometimes the hardest thing about dinnertime is deciding what to have. One method for simplifying this daily deliberation is to designate a type of meal for each night of the week. For instance, Monday is always chicken night, Tuesday is pasta, Wednesday is seafood, Thursday is beef, and Friday is pizza. Having a starting point often makes it easier to brainstorm for specific meal ideas.

Use Make-Ahead Meals: There are many ways to do this. You can form a Make-Ahead Meal Group, where each group member makes a designated number of meals, freezes the individual meals, and then gets together and exchanges them so everyone comes home with different meals to keep in the freezer to feed their family throughout the month. If a Make-Ahead Meal Group is not for you, double or triple the recipes in this book and freeze them for your own family. See the Make-Ahead Meal Group chapter to learn more and to get started on really planning ahead!

Implement Kid Suggestions

To find out how children are affected by family dinnertime, I decided to go right to the source. I interviewed many children to get these insightful answers about the importance and significance of sharing the family dinner table. Here are a few.

Q. What is your favorite thing that your mom makes you for dinner?

Kyra R., age 12—Tacos

Kuen R., age 11—Italian chicken

Tatem R., age 8—Porcupine meatballs. Yum!

Bryson R., age 5—Rice

Eli E., age 8 —Spaghetti

Abby E., age 5—Salad

Emma E., age 7—Lasagna

Brigham E., age 13—Chicken noodle soup and lemon bars

Lincoln E., age 10—Chicken Alfredo

Tiberius P., age 4—Salmon and chicken nuggets

Thadeus P., age 6—Pizza

Hannah T., age 4—Beans

Taylor T., age 11—Turkey tetrazzini

Michaela H., age 9—Bow ties and shrimp

Ericka H., age 4—Corn dogs. Yum!

Malorie H., age 5—French fries and sandwiches

Alex H., age 8—Chicken on a bone

Jaxon E., age 7—Anything and everything!

Cora G., age 8—Omelets

Isabella D., age 4—Quesadillas

Gavin E., age 2—Noodles

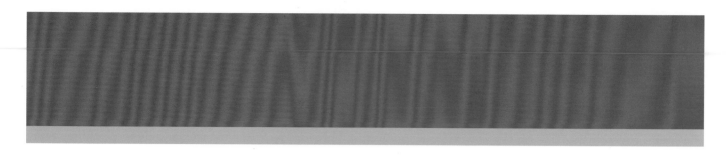

Q. What is your least favorite thing that your mom makes for dinner?

Kyra R., age 12—Lasagna

Kuen R., age 11—Everything that contains ground beef.

Tatem R., age 8—Chicken macaroni bake

Bryson R., age 5—Chicken

Grace T., age 7—Fireman food (chili)

Emily H., age 10—The one casserole she makes with broccoli.

Megan H., age 6—Potatoes

Tiberius P., age 4—I don't like stuff Mom cooks, just what Dad cooks.

Eli E., age 8—That green stuff.

Elise E., age 10—Squash and zucchini

Aurora G., age 10—Mashed squash

Isabella D., age 4—Spinach

Olvia E., age 4—Celery

Gavin E., age 2—Carrots

Q. Why is it important to eat dinner together as a family?

Eli E., age 8—To build relationships.

Emma E., age 5—To talk together.

Emma M., age 8—Spend time as a family.

Bryson R., age 5—To play games.

Olivia M., age 4—Dinner helps your body get more energy.

William M., age 10—It helps you love your family more.

Eli E., age 8—It's the best thing ever, unless Mom makes that green stuff!

Chase K., age 6—To get healthy.

Taylor T., age 11—You can talk over problems.

Hannah T., age 4—Because!

Haydon T., age 8—To spend time together.

Isabelle H., age 4—Cause I love dinner.

Tatem R., age 8—To have fun.

Emily H., age 10—To be together as a family for at least 10 minutes.

Thadeus P., age 6—Because it's fun!

Zoee B., age 8—Because we're a family and we love each other.

Malorie H., age 5—It helps your body be happy.

Alex H., age 8—You actually be together forever.

Jaden E., age 13—Family planning.

Isabella D., age 4—Sitting together.

Olivia E., age 4—Because we love each other.

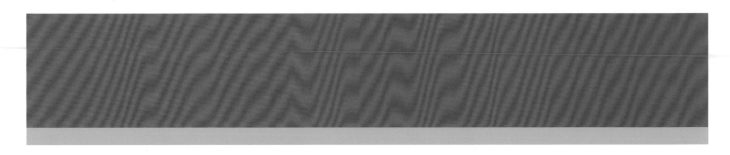

Q. What does your mom do best?

Meaghan H., age 6—Loves us and takes care of us.

Michaela H., age 9—Taking care of us and making good food.

Erika H., age 4—(She whispers to Mom, "Give me a clue!") Makes good food!

Emma M., age 8—Setting the table, decorating, sewing, and tucking me in bed.

Olivia M., age 4—Doing dishes and helping with piano.

William M., age 10—Helping and having fun.

Bryson R., age 5—Go to Disneyland.

Chalet T., age 14—Makes sure we have a healthy dinner.

Hannah T., age 4—Buys strawberries!

Quincy S., age 6—Works in the garden.

Tatem R., age 8—Lets us sleep in her bed.

Hayden T., age 8—Makes sure we don't eat a lot of sugar.

Jaden E., age 13—Loves and takes care of us (and everyone else)!

Kyra R., age 12—Cook.

Tiberius P., age 4—Laundry.

Kuen R., age 11—Clean.

Aurora G., age 10—Loving us.

Cora G., age 8—Art.

Isabella D., age 4—Put us to bed.

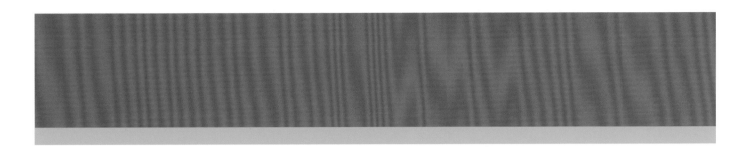

Gavin E., age 2—Tickle me.

Olivia E., age 4—Lets me paint.

Chase K., age 6—Lets me go play with my friends.

Q. What would you miss out on if you didn't eat dinner together as a family?

Chalet T., age 14—You wouldn't be a very close family.

Mckayla T., age 16—You wouldn't know what is going on with everyone.

Hayden T., age 8—Dinner!

Madi N., age 8—Prayer.

Tiberius P., age 4—My favorite person to talk to: Daddy.

Keller B., age 4—I would be hungry!

Dallin H., age 12—Having someone to talk to.

Elise E., age 10—Inspiration.

Jaden E., age 13—Love and support.

Bryson R., age 5—Eating.

Michaela H., age 9—Homemade desserts!

Erika H., age 4—Peach smoothies! Yum!

Cora G., age 8—Mommy and Daddy!

Olivia E., age 4—Then we would be hungry.

Chase K., age 6—Eating my favorite things.

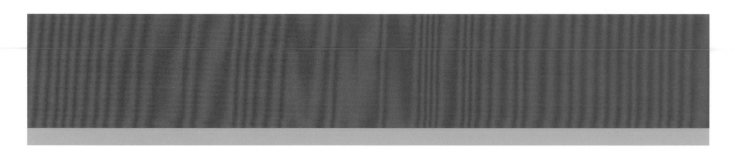

Q. What do you talk about or do at the dinner table?

William M., age 10—We talk about stuff and play word games.

Emma M., age 8—Sometimes if we like our dinner, it is really quiet.

Olivia M., age 4—What we have to do at school.

Erika H., age 4—I like to sing!

Michaela H., age 9—Animal facts. I teach them all I know about animals.

Meaghan H., age 6—School and our day.

Eli E., age 8—We plan the next day.

Chase Q., age 9—Sometimes we make fun of each other.

Casey Q., age 13—Yeah, my dad says I chew like a cow!

Sara H., age 10—Talk about our highs and lows for the day.

Olivia E., age 4—About chewing.

Bryson R., age 6—Your good things and bad things. The things you hate and love.

Q. If you could describe your family dinnertime in one word, what would it be?

Hannah T., age 4—Eating!

Taylor T., age 11—Happy (glad there's food!)

Megan H., age 6—Special

Madi N., age 8—Fun

Emily H., age 10—Happy

Chase Q., age 8—Talk

Casey Q., age 13—Fun

Zoee B., age 8—Yummy

Jaxon E., age 7—Awesome!

Elise E., age 10—Fun!

Jaden E., age 13—Heavenly! (Coming from a 13-year-old boy!)

Aurora G., age 10—Fun!

Gavin D., age 2—Fun!

Olivia E., age 4—Nice.

Kyra R., age 12—Crazy!

The importance of eating dinner together goes beyond statistics and conversation—it's love, time, relationships, support, and of course, peach smoothies! Children feel the effects of our efforts in making dinnertime special; they notice and care. And as you listen to your children's suggestions, you'll find ways to make dinnertime fun, meaningful, and special for them even if it feels crazy and overwhelming for you. Keep it up! Just remember—kids do not like green stuff in their food. (But keep that up too!)

Laugh Together

All right, you've planned ahead and gotten a healthy meal on the table and actually gotten your entire family sitting in one place at one time for dinner. Quite the task, isn't it? The next question is, What do we do now? First, let's answer the question, What do we not do now? Remember, your goal is to spend more than 35 minutes a week in active conversation with your children. Since this time is crucial, make it count. This should not be family meeting time. This is the time for you and your family to visit, have conversations, get to know each other, find out about each other's day, and laugh together. Make this a positive experience, or they will dread it—and this will detract from the effort of making family meals happen.

Here are a few ideas to get the ball rolling on how to make family dinner a pleasant experience:

- **Take turns telling jokes:** You could even have a joke book handy.

- **A great and a grumble:** Have each person take turns telling one great thing and one not-so-great thing that happened that day. This will give you an opportunity to see what makes your children happy and maybe even some things that are bothering them. This also provides an opportunity for the entire family to help problem-solve together if there are grumbles like someone bullying your child at school or not doing well on a test. You could discuss ways to fix the problems and make other siblings aware of things going on at school where you cannot be all the time. You may find that you learn more this way than by just asking, "How was your day?"

- **"I'm going to the grocery store" game:** To play this game, each person adds on an item in alphabetical order that you could buy at the grocery store. For instance, the first person might say, "I'm going to the grocery store, and I'm going to buy an apple." The next person could say, "I'm going to the grocery store, and I'm going to buy an apple and a banana." Go through the whole alphabet until someone forgets the order or an item. That person is then out, and you continue on with the game.

- **Pass-along story:** Have everyone add one sentence to a story. You can make this as long as you would like. It will make you get creative, make you laugh together, and can create some fun family inside jokes.

- **"I spy" game:** Choose an item in the room or on the dinner table and provide a hint about what letter it starts with or what color it is—"I spy something green"—and then let each person take a turn guessing what the item is and asking questions about it.

- **"What's missing?" game:** One person closes his eyes and someone takes an item off the table. When the person opens his eyes, he must figure out what is missing from the table.

- **Share family memories:** Have each person share a favorite memory. This is a great one for parents to participate in. Your children love to hear stories from your childhood. It's also a way to find out what makes great memories for your children.

- **Talk about your favorite teacher:** Have each person share who his favorite teacher is and why. This will give you an idea of the kind of people your children look up to.

- **Sing a song one word at a time:** Choose a song that everyone knows, such as "Twinkle, Twinkle Little Star." Go around the table and let each person sing one word each until you complete the song.

- **Eat without utensils:** Instead of utensils, give each person a pair of rubber gloves. You can even ditch the plates as well and put spaghetti right on a plastic tablecloth. Twenty years from now, your kids will still be talking about what a cool mom they had!

- **Tie wrists together:** Have fun and teach kids teamwork at the same time!

- **Share embarrassing moments:** Let everyone share their most embarrassing moments. This may surprise you!

- **Be kings and queens:** Let everyone be kings and queens for a night. Emphasize manners, and drink with pinkies up. You could even appoint someone as the servant—preferably not Mom!

- **Share your dream vacation:** Let everyone share their dream vacation. Where would they go? What would they see, do, and eat?

- **Share what life will be like when you grow up:** Ask everyone what they expect life to be like when they grow up. This could include what they want to do for a living, what cars will be like, what houses will look like, what kind of person they will marry, how many kids they will have, and where they will live. This is the kind of stuff you'll want to write down later so years from now you can read this back to them!

- **Spotlight each person:** Choose one person to be in the spotlight, and let everyone at the table say one thing that makes this person special. You can go around the table until everyone has had a chance to be in the spotlight. This will help siblings realize that there are actually good things about every person, even though they may have to think for a minute!

Make and Record Memories

Do you have a story about a certain recipe? Maybe it's just a favorite birthday dinner your mom would make especially for you or the rolls that your grandma made every Thanksgiving. Some recipe stories are funny, and some take you down memory lane. Make sure you record your special family stories! Also, I would love for you to share your recipes and stories at onthegocookbook.blogspot.com and join other families in our quest to bring families back to the table.

Some of my favorite recipe stories come from my childhood, and some are from my own little family, or even friends.

One day, I was sitting on my front porch enjoying a book when the little boy from across the street ran out of his house and enthusiastically yelled to his big brother, "Nick, Nick!" I thought to myself, *Boy, he must have found out they were going to Disneyland or something!* He continued to run toward his brother as he was jumping for joy! "Nick, Mom made corn bread for dinner!" They gave each other a high-five and together ran home, both jumping for joy and hollering, "Corn bread, corn bread!" I thought, *That must be SOME corn bread.* I called the next day to get that corn bread recipe from their mom, and it is now called Jump for Joy Corn Bread.

Another story from my family is the day my mom made our family's favorite "Frozen Raspberry Dessert." This was an especially popular one with my dad. My younger brother was not home at the time, so we saved him the last piece. My dad's mouth watered for hours knowing that it was in the freezer untouched. When my brother finally returned home, my dad offered him five dollars for the coveted piece of dessert. My brother accepted happily, and now it is called The $5 Dessert.

There are even stories in my family about not-so-loved recipes, such as the time my aunt made stew at our home, and for some unknown reason, she put peanut butter in it. We all thought it tasted a little odd, and we asked her what was in it. She fessed up, and we still, twenty-five years later, talk about peanut butter stew.

Another not-so-tasty story is the time I was expecting my fifth child. I was so ready to have this baby, and I had heard that eggplant has the same hormone that is released in your body to put you into labor. So I had my parents over for dinner and I made eggplant Parmesan. I had never had eggplant before, but I was determined to go into labor. I was told you have to eat a lot of eggplant to make it work. I didn't care for it, but I gagged it down anyway. Later, my mom confessed that she had to gag it down also. She was nice enough to say that the eggplant must have not been a good one, not that the cook wasn't a good one! Needless to say, I was still pregnant for two more weeks.

These are recipe stories that have made great memories for our family. Many of these recipes are from friends and family and have become our family memories. I hope these stories will get you remembering, compiling, sharing, and recording your own recipe stories. And feel free to share your recipe stories at www.onthegocookbook.blogspot.com.

These are the times you want to remember. As you make dinnertime special, you will hear some things come out of those little ones' mouths. If you're like me, the next day you'll say, "Now what was that funny thing he said?" Like the dinner where my seven-year-old son asked, "Mom, did you have Heelys when you were a kid?" I said no, and he responded, "Oh yeah, because that was back in the pioneer times, huh?"

Memories are often made over food, and one day you may see the impact your dinner traditions have made on your children. We have Sunday dinner as soon as we can get home from church and get it on the table. Sometimes that may even be more like lunchtime, but it is still called "Sunday dinner." My kids couldn't figure that out. They would ask, "So is this lunch or dinner?" I finally started calling it "linner." They now know that I only make one meal on Sunday and the rest is FFY (Fend For Yourself). We often go to my parents' house for Sunday "linner." One year for Christmas, my ten-year-old daughter wrote this poem for my mom:

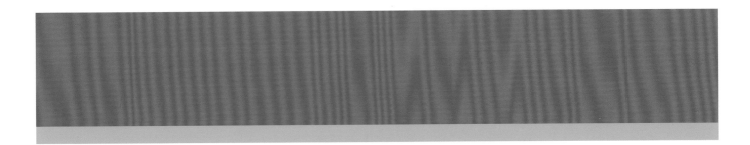

Grandparents are nice
Like sugar and spice.
They feed you dinner,
Lunch, and linner.
I know they are old
And can't be sold
But they are still good to hold!

Then there are the memorable events, like the time I had my brother and his family over for dinner. We had lasagna (Mom's recipe, of course) and fettuccine Alfredo. My eighteen-month-old son started rubbing his nose and acting strangely. We were all staring at him, not knowing what to think, when all of a sudden he sneezed and a long fettuccine noodle shot out of his nose and across the room. We will never look at fettuccine the same way!

And then there was the time when I was a teenager, and my mom invited my boyfriend to stay for dinner. A few minutes into the meal, I started choking, and my dad had to give me the Heimlich maneuver. I won't forget these events any time soon, but don't trust your memory. Write it down! Here are some spaces provided for just that purpose.

Date ——————————

———————————————————————
———————————————————————
———————————————————————

Date ——————————

———————————————————————
———————————————————————
———————————————————————

Date _____

_____
_____
_____

Date _____

_____
_____
_____

Date _____

_____
_____
_____

Date _____

_____
_____
_____

Date _____

_____
_____
_____

Date _____

_____

_____

_____

Date _____

_____

_____

_____

Date _____

_____

_____

_____

Date _____

_____

_____

_____

Date _____

_____

_____

_____

All About Make-Ahead Meals

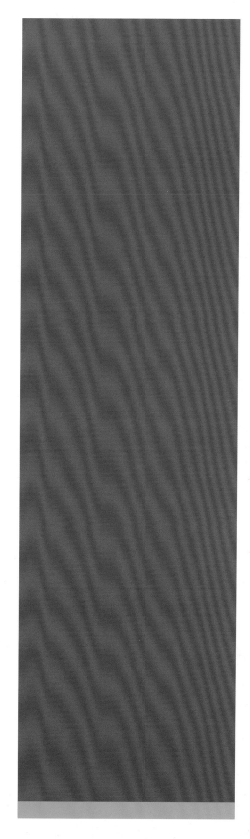

Introduction

It's one of those days. You know—*those* days. The phone is ringing off the hook, the kids need help with their homework, your husband is working late, you have a PTA meeting in an hour, and you still have to pick the kids up from soccer practice. Then you think about dinner. Dinner? Okay, here are the quick and easy choices: pizza, pizza, or pizza. Okay, kids . . . how about pizza?

As you fall into bed later that night and analyze your day, you realize that all was running smoothly, one challenge at a time, until 5:00 p.m. Dinnertime came and you weren't prepared, so everything else seemed to fall apart. Does it seem to be this way more often than not? Do you want it to be different?

This book is tailored to the mom who does it all—the mom with a busy life and busy children but who wants to have peaceful, fulfilling family time every night at the dinner table; the mom who wants to feed her family home-cooked meals but wants to spend less time planning and preparing those meals.

Whether you want to start a Make-Ahead Meal Group or just prepare Make-Ahead Meals for your own family, this book is the tool to help you achieve that goal. It assists you in planning and preparing Make-Ahead Meals that have been tried and tested by actual Make-Ahead Meal Groups. We've picked only the best meals for you and your family.

Good luck in your endeavors to simplify life, save time and money, enjoy more family time, make some great friends, and be treated to a variety of delicious home-cooked meals.

What Is a Make-Ahead Meal Group?

A Make-Ahead Meal Group is a group of people who prepare and freeze a designated number of servings for the same meal of their choice in the convenience of their own home. Then they get together to exchange dishes so that each member of the group takes home that same number of various meals. This process is designed to save time, money, and stress by spending one afternoon making one meal in bulk rather than spending the time every night to prepare a home-cooked meal for your family. This book will give you the tricks of the trade—along with many tried and true recipes to help you simplify dinnertime in your own home.

How to Start Your Own Make-Ahead Meal Group

Invite people to join your group:

Think of all the moms you know who could use a little simplifying in their lives—maybe your neighbor, friend, sister-in-law, or fellow soccer moms. Think of those moms who are dependable, good cooks, and have healthy homes (clean kitchen habits). These are the type of people you should look for so that you feel good about where your meals are coming from. You may also suggest that your members get a food handler's permit. It isn't necessary, but it's a good idea for food safety. (Call your local health department for information.)

Make some rules and guidelines:

It is important that everyone in your group knows exactly what is expected of them so that everyone can do her part. (See page 31 for sample guidelines.) You'll want to have a meeting before your group starts so that everyone can decide what works best for your specific group. The issues to address are:

- **How many people** each meal must feed. For example, many groups set the amount at 6 adult servings, and if the meal is in a casserole dish, require that the dish be 9×13 inches in size. For those families that don't eat quite that much, the excess is perfect for leftovers and to send with your husband to work the next day.

- **Decide what preferences** you will cater to. For instance, some groups prefer boneless, skinless chicken breasts. Also, you will need to address food allergies. Many groups find it is easier to not have any food allergy guidelines. However, if the majority of group members prefer low-fat or all-chicken meals, then make it a group requirement.

- **Decide a time** and place to exchange. In case someone can't make it to the exchange on the specified day, it is helpful to make the exchange at the house of a member who has extra freezer space. Then those who can't make it to the exchange can deliver their meals the day before and have somewhere to keep them frozen until the other members pick up the meals. Coolers with ice also work well if any group members will be picking up the meals shortly after the exchange.

• **Decide when, where,** and how often to exchange meals. Choosing a specific day of each month will help your members always know when it is coming and plan around it. Exchanges can be bi-monthly or however often your group wants it to be. Choosing a date such as the second Friday of every month is often easier than, for example, the 10th of each month, so that you avoid hitting the weekends.

• **Set an approximate** price range. Otherwise, someone may spend $30 on her meals and someone else may spend $150. A good average is $75. It is feasible to spend less, especially if you watch the sales, but encourage your members not to go over the budget.

• **Have group members** bring copies of their recipes to each exchange. A full sheet of paper can be kept in a binder specifically for Make-Ahead Meal recipes. Or exchange 3×5 recipe cards to fit in your recipe file. Do whatever works best for group members. Each member should put her name and phone number on her recipe in case other members have questions about it. Side dish suggestions are a helpful addition to each recipe.

• **Decide who is** in charge. Your group may want to take turns making reminder calls. Some groups may not even need reminder calls, but it is often appreciated. Most groups choose one person as the president, so to say, and she does all the reminding and finds people to fill vacant spots. The president could change every year if desired.

After the meeting, send group members a welcome letter or email that includes all the guidelines decided by the group. Make sure each member receives one. This is especially nice for new members who join later. See a sample guideline letter on page 31.

Welcome to the Make-Ahead Meal Group!

Here are the guidelines:

• **You will** be required to make and freeze 10 meals to exchange with our group.

• **Try to** spend around or below $75 for all costs.

• **Your meal** should feed 6 adults. (If the item is in a pan, please use a 9×13.)

• **You will** need to package your meal either in freezer bags or disposable aluminum pans.

• **Write on** your packaging with permanent marker what the meal is, the basic instructions, and the date (example: Chicken Casserole, 350° for 30 min, 02/02/10). You will probably have to pull the meal out of the freezer ahead of time so that it can thaw. Write the cook time that should be used once the meal is thawed.

• **Please only** make meals that you and your family have tried and enjoy. Don't experiment on the group!

• **If you** are stumped about what to cook and what freezes well, there are two great books that have all the tips and recipes that you'll need. They are called *Girlfriends on the Go: A Busy Mom's Guide to Make-Ahead Meals* and *Families on the Go* by Suzie Roberts.

• **Type up** each of your recipes on a full sheet of paper as well as suggestions for what vegetables or side dishes to serve with the meal. We want to put each recipe in its own sheet protector so that we can put together a binder specifically for Make-Ahead Meal recipes. Also, write your name on the recipe page so that we remember who made the meal.

• **We want** everyone to have fun. Obviously your family is not going to love every meal, but hopefully they will enjoy the majority and that will make it all worthwhile. The most important thing is to take some stress out of your day so that you can spend more time with your family doing fun things, not cooking and cleaning!

• **Also, pay** attention to your grocery and dining-out budget so that you can see the money you've saved.

Our next meal exchange will be on _____ at _____'s house at _____.

Her address is _____.

Please bring your meals already frozen. Plan ahead! If you cannot make it to the exchange, please drop off the meals in a cooler (with ice) prior to the exchange. If you are not prepared, each person will keep her meal until you deliver your meal and pick up the others from each group member. We will meet every second Friday to exchange and talk about our dishes. It shouldn't take more than 45 minutes.

Please call if you have any questions!

Frequently Asked Questions about Make-Ahead Meal Groups

How long does it take to prepare 10 meals?

It depends on the meal. It usually takes 2–4 hours. We have found that it works best in shifts. For instance, one day you can cook all the meat and the next day assemble the rest. It may sound like a long time, but those ten days that you don't have to take the time and have the mess of preparing meals makes it worth it. With good planning, you can save time and frustration by preparing your meals when your kids are asleep or at school.

How does a Make-Ahead Meal Group save you money?

Let me count the ways . . .

- **First, you** go to the grocery store less often. Do you ever go to the store for milk and bread and end up coming out with 10 other items you didn't need? The less often you visit the store, the less money you will spend.

- **Your shopping** list for Make-Ahead Meals is simple. You don't need a list of items for 10 different meals. Instead, you buy 10 of the same thing. Simple is good.

- **You can** plan your meals around what's on sale. If ground beef is on sale, choose a recipe for that month that calls for ground beef.

- **You'll eat** out less. Fridays and Saturdays are great times for Make-Ahead Meals because those are usually the days that you don't feel like cooking. Pull a meal out of the freezer on days you know you won't have time to cook.

- **You have** less waste. Since you don't purchase ingredients for several different meals, perishable ingredients don't go bad before you have a chance to use them.

- **You can** purchase items in bulk. Watch those sales or shop at a warehouse store (like Costco). It's cheaper and leaves less packaging to throw away.

What if someone quits?

If someone quits, try to fill the spot as soon as possible. If you are not able to fill that spot in time for the next exchange, you have several options:

1. On the exchange day, tell everyone in your group to take their extra meal home with them.

2. Have everyone exchange their extra meal among themselves so that they take two of another meal home instead of two of their own.

3. Give the extra meals to someone who needs it that month, such as someone who just had surgery or had a baby or someone whose spouse is on military duty.

4. Another option is to have a substitute that is willing to participate when someone is unable to do it. (Continued on next page.)

How does a Make-Ahead Meal Group save you time?

If you spend 4 hours making 10 meals, including prep and cleanup, you will save yourself as many as 16 hours a month. How? If you were to make a meal every night for 10 nights, you would take approximately 15 minutes to decide what you'll have, 30 minutes to run to the store to get the ingredients you're missing, and 45 minutes to chop, boil, brown, marinate, simmer, and assemble. Then there are all the dishes, pots, bowls, cutting boards, utensils, and appliances you used in the preparation process that you need to wash, dry, and put away. That takes you at least another 20 minutes. As you are doing all of this, of course there are at least 15 minutes of interruptions. You don't always realize that it takes so much time to prepare a meal every night, but you will realize the extra time on those 10 nights that you don't have to.

How many people should be in the group?

Ten is usually the best number. Each group can decide for itself how many meals to make. Most groups find that ten meals are a good amount to exchange each month. That way, you can still fix your family favorites on some days and have leftovers other days. I personally have found that the best use of the meals is to eat them on your busiest days. Maybe Tuesdays are T-ball games and piano lessons. Use a Make-Ahead Meal on those days. I almost always use Make-Ahead Meals on Fridays since that is the day I have found that I don't feel like cooking and would usually order pizza. For many people, Sundays are good for Make-Ahead Meals because it takes less effort to put a nice Sunday dinner on the table—and much less cleanup.

What if we have picky eaters?

Obviously there are going to be some meals that members of your family just don't like. Before I started the Make-Ahead Meal Group, I could count on one hand the things my six-year-old son would eat. However, I felt it was important for him to learn to try new things and believed that if he would try new things, he would like them. Since we always had a variety of food and didn't always have the same old meals that I knew all my kids would eat, he had to learn to try many new things. A year later, he would eat any kind of chicken and some casseroles. For me, that has been the biggest reward from the Make-Ahead Meal Group. Since then, I have had a one-year-old who loves any food I put in front of him. I believe that this acceptance of foods is a result from having a variety of meals from a young age.

What are other benefits of a Make-Ahead Meal Group?

• **Someone else's** cooking: Sometimes food just tastes better when someone else prepares it—not because you're not a good cook, but because you don't have to cook it.

• **Variety:** You don't always have the same old meals. Of course, your family has their favorites, and the days you don't use a Make-Ahead Meal are perfect for those family favorites. People often find that meals they'd never considered making have become a new favorite.

• **Sick Days:** Mom doesn't get a day off when she's sick—it's nice to have one less thing to do on those days.

• **Dad's turn** to cook: Dad will love the Make-Ahead Meals on those nights he's in charge. With the instructions written right on the package, he can just put a meal in the oven when it's his turn to cook.

• **Serving others:** When a friend or a loved one is having a hard time, it's nice to have a meal that you can easily share. Some people in our Make-Ahead Meal Group choose to make an extra meal each month, and we get together and take the extra meals to someone in need that month, such as a family whose mom or dad is on military duty, a mom who just had a baby, someone having financial troubles, someone who has had a death in the family or a serious illness, and so forth. It's interesting how a few meals can take a large burden off someone in need.

What is the best way to thaw our Make-Ahead Meals?

For best results, let frozen meals thaw in the refrigerator for 24 hours. For those of us who don't think that far in advance, here are some other tips:

• **If cooking** directly from frozen, as a rule of thumb, bump up the temperature 50° higher than the recipe states, and double the time. Generally, this is ample time to cook your frozen meal. You will need to check it periodically to make sure you are on target.

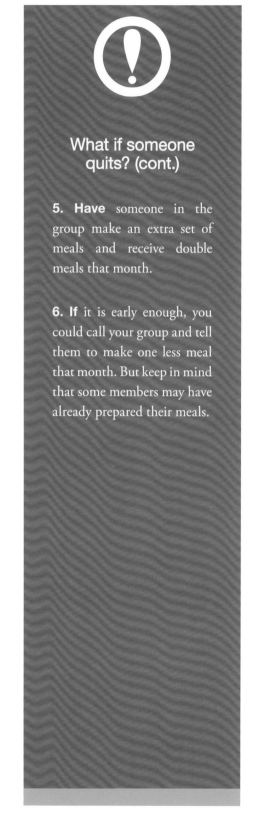

What if someone quits? (cont.)

5. Have someone in the group make an extra set of meals and receive double meals that month.

6. If it is early enough, you could call your group and tell them to make one less meal that month. But keep in mind that some members may have already prepared their meals.

Flash Freezing

Sometimes you will need to flash freeze items such as taquitos or chicken nuggets —anything you will put in a freezer bag in which you don't want individual items to stick together.

To flash freeze, place the items on a cookie sheet and put it in the freezer. As soon as they are no longer soft to the touch they are ready to be placed in a bag and returned to the freezer.

• **If you** will be out of the house all day, a slow cooker meal is perfect. You can put it in your slow cooker in the morning and it will be ready at dinnertime. If there are no slow cooker meals in your freezer, your time-delay cook on your oven is also a wonderful tool. Place your meal in the oven at your convenience. Set your bake time about 1½ times the amount called for in the recipe, and set your temperature 25°–50° higher. Your meal will have time to partially thaw in the oven until it starts to cook at the designated time. What a good feeling to walk in to the scent of a nice home-cooked meal after a hard day's work.

Make-Ahead Meal Tips

As you are trying to make your life simpler, read all the tips I've learned through years of experience with Make-Ahead Meals. This will save you from having to experiment yourself. I have made these recipes as simple as possible to make it less time consuming and more productive for you. Remember, the people who need Make-Ahead Meals are the ones who don't have time for the small details, just the cold, hard meal!

What to freeze your meals in:

Freezer Bags:

- **If at** all possible, freeze your meals in freezer bags. They are the cheapest way to go. Many soups, sauces, and non-layered casseroles can be frozen in a gallon-size freezer bag.

- **Squeeze as** much air out of the bag as you can. The less air, the less freezer taste and freezer burn your meal will have.

- **Label the** freezer bag *before* you fill it and freeze it.

- **Once filled,** lay your bag flat in the freezer. It will freeze quicker that way and take up less room in the freezer. Don't stack meals on top of each other until after they are frozen so that they can freeze properly in the middle.

Disposable Pans:

- **Disposable aluminum** pans work great for anything that can't be put in a freezer bag.

- **Make sure** you cover the dish tightly with foil. You may also wish to use a double layer of foil or freezer foil to protect your meals even more. If the meal is tomato based, cover with plastic wrap and then foil. The acid from the tomatoes can eat away the foil.

- **You can** purchase disposable aluminum pans in bulk at wholesale stores. They end up being about 25 cents apiece. It is so nice to just throw away the mess, instead of soaking and scrubbing a pan.

Foods that may not freeze well:

• **If you** are making a meal that uses flour tortillas, such as enchiladas, freeze the enchiladas separate from the sauce. Put the sauce in a quart-size freezer bag and freeze along with the meal. Otherwise, your tortillas may get very mushy.

• **If your** meal calls for cooked rice or pasta, undercook it, or it will get mushy from freezing and thawing.

• **Raw potatoes** or squashes do not freeze well. If you are using potatoes or vegetables that need to be cooked before freezing, undercook them so they don't get mushy. Potatoes tend to get mushy anyway. If possible, replace potatoes with frozen hash browns, which have been commercially prepared for freezing.

(Continued on next page.)

Cooking Meat in Bulk

When you are preparing meals for a group, it is easier to cook your meat in bulk. Here are some ways to simplify this process.

• **Ground Beef:** Crumble 3 to 4 lbs. on a large cookie sheet with sides. Place in a preheated oven at 425° and bake for 20 minutes or until meat is no longer pink. Make sure you use extra-lean or extra-extra lean for this process unless you use a casserole dish with taller sides. Otherwise the grease may drip over the edge. Pull out of the oven when done. Place meat in a colander under hot water. Rinse off extra grease as you use a spatula to crumble the meat.

• **Another way** to cook ground beef in bulk is to place in boiling water in a stockpot and boil until no longer pink. Then, rinse in a colander as well.

• **Chicken:** A large slow cooker will do 10–12 chicken breasts at a time. Place them in the slow cooker with 1 cup of water and cook on medium or high for 2–3 hours (longer if you want to shred it–shorter if you want it whole or to cube it). You can also cook it on low overnight in a slow cooker. Anything you can do while you sleep is a great way to multi-task! Such a motherly thing to do!

• **Roasts:** Use a large slow cooker for 1–2 roasts, or even better, use a roaster oven to do 5–6 at a time. Cook on medium overnight. When you wake up, they are ready to shred.

Make-Ahead Meal Icons

The exclamation mark icon will alert you to tips and tricks that make freezing meals easier.

The shopping cart icon will show you a list of ingredients you will need in order to make a Make-Ahead Meal for 10 families.

The snowflake icon appears with each recipe to give you directions for freezing the meal.

Foods that may not freeze well (cont.):

• **Sauces with** sour cream, cream cheese, and cream freeze fine. Depending on the ratio of cream in the sauce, you may need to whisk sauce after re-heating since it may separate slightly after freezing.

The Process

Yes, there can be some method to the madness.

1. After you decide on the meal you want to prepare, check your pantry. Most of the main ingredients called for will probably need to be purchased, but you may already have the spices or other small ingredients. However, don't assume you have enough. You may think you definitely have garlic powder, but if your recipe calls for 1 teaspoon, you will need 10 teaspoons. Nothing is worse than being up to your elbows assembling 10 meals and realizing that you're short one ingredient.

2. After shopping and making sure you have all the ingredients, decide on the pre-meal details. Is it a meal in which the meat needs to be browned, cooked, shredded, or cubed? See our section on cooking meat in bulk for tips on streamlining that process.

3. When you're getting ready to prepare the meals, get everything out and set it in sections around your kitchen, placing each ingredient in order as it is used in the recipe.

> • **Open all** the items in cans or packages before you start. It saves time and mess. Also, have packaging labeled and ready to fill, so that once you're finished assembling, you can place the prepared meal directly into the freezer.

4. You can choose one of two ways to assemble. If the meal has to be mixed in a bowl, it is easier to mix each meal separately, and then place it in the appropriate freezing container.

> • **For instance,** if you are making a soup, go down the line and place all the ingredients in the bowl, mix up, and pour into a freezer bag. If it is a soup that has to be cooked first, you could possibly double or triple the batch in a stockpot to save time. If your meal is something such as a layered casserole, you may want to do it assembly style.

> • **Place all** the pans out on the table. Prepare the first layer for all 10 meals, place in pan, and move on to the second ingredient. This is very quick and easy.

5. Do not stack meals on top of each other in the freezer before they are completely frozen. Stacking makes it hard for the center to freeze in a timely manner.

Make-Ahead Meal Recipes

These recipes have been compiled from actual Make-Ahead Meal Groups. They are the tried-and-true family favorites of Make-Ahead Meal Group members and have since become some of our family favorites. I hope they will soon become some of your family favorites. Whether you are preparing Make-Ahead Meals for your own family, forming a Make-Ahead Meal Group, or just need some new ideas for dinner, these recipes are sure to please!

Beef Recipes

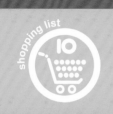
- 20 lbs. beef flank steak

- 5 cups soy sauce

- 1¼ cups molasses

- 7 Tbsp. ground mustard

- 3 Tbsp. + 1 tsp.
  ground ginger

- 5 tsp. garlic powder

Grilled Steak Skewers

Kids love anything on a stick!

2 lbs. beef flank steak (or substitute sirloin
   to save money)
½ cup soy sauce
¼ cup water
2 Tbsp. molasses
2 tsp. ground mustard
1 tsp. ground ginger
½ tsp. garlic powder

Ask your butcher to slice the steak into ¼-inch slices at the time of purchase. If you do it yourself, freeze for an hour and then slice for easier cutting. Combine all the ingredients in a gallon-size freezer bag. Seal the bag and coat the steak. If freezing, see directions below. Otherwise, soak skewers in water so they don't catch fire on the grill, and then thread meat ribbon-style on skewers. Grill over medium heat for 3–4 minutes on each side or until done.

Freezing directions: Freeze in the freezer bag. Include skewers with this meal.

Hamburger Casserole

A fabulous taste, surprisingly easy!

1½ lbs. ground beef
½ cup chopped onion
1 (12-oz.) pkg. wide egg noodles
1 (12-oz.) can corn
1 can cream of mushroom soup
1 cup sour cream
¾ tsp. salt
¼ tsp. accent (optional)
¼ tsp. pepper
1 cup bread crumbs
1 Tbsp. butter, melted

Brown ground beef and onion. Drain. If freezing, see directions below. Otherwise, cook noodles according to package directions and drain. Mix together all ingredients except bread crumbs. Place mixture in a 9×13 pan. Top with bread crumbs. Bake at 350 degrees for 30 minutes.

Freezing directions: Only cook the noodles for half the time called for in the directions. Mix all ingredients except bread crumbs. Place mixture in a disposable pan. Top with bread crumbs. Cover with foil and freeze.

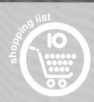

shopping list

- 15 lbs. ground beef

- 5 medium onions

- 10 (12-oz.) pkgs. wide egg noodles

- 10 (12-oz.) cans corn

- 10 cans cream of mushroom soup

- 5 pints sour cream

- Abt. 3 Tbsp. salt

- Abt. 1 Tbsp. accent

- Abt. 1 Tbsp. pepper

- 1 cup + 2 Tbsp. butter

- 10 cups bread crumbs

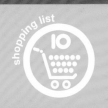

shopping list

- 15 lbs. ground beef

- 10 medium onions

- 3 Tbsp. + 1 tsp. garlic powder

- 5 tsp. garlic salt

- 10 (14-oz.) jars spaghetti sauce

- 10 (6-oz.) cans tomato paste

- 10 (12-oz.) bags small shell pasta

- 10 (16-oz.) tubs sour cream

- 5 cups Parmesan cheese

- 7½ lbs. shredded mozzarella cheese

Lasagna and Shells Casserole

This kid-friendly version of lasagna will please kids and adults alike!

1½ lbs. ground beef, browned
1 medium onion, chopped
1 tsp. garlic powder
½ tsp. garlic salt
1 (14-oz.) jar spaghetti sauce
1 (6-oz.) can tomato paste
12 oz. small shell pasta
1 (16-oz.) tub sour cream
½ cup Parmesan cheese
3 cups shredded mozzarella cheese

In a skillet, combine browned ground beef, chopped onion, garlic powder, garlic salt, spaghetti sauce, and tomato paste. Simmer over medium heat for 15–20 minutes. Cook pasta according to package directions. (If freezing, do not cook pasta.) Place half of the pasta in the bottom of a 9 × 13 pan. Top with half of the meat sauce. Spread 1 cup sour cream on top and sprinkle with ¼ cup Parmesan cheese. Then sprinkle with 1½ cups mozzarella cheese. Repeat layers. If freezing, see directions below. Otherwise, cover and bake at 375 degrees for 45 minutes. Uncover and bake for 10 more minutes.

Freezing directions: There is no need to cook pasta if freezing this recipe. Place casserole in a disposable pan. Cover with plastic wrap and then aluminum foil. Freeze. Make sure to remove plastic wrap and re-cover with foil before baking.

Pizza and Pasta Bake

Combine the favorites of pizza and pasta, and kids will go wild!

1 (16-oz.) pkg. spiral pasta
1 lb. ground beef, browned
1 onion, chopped
1 tsp. salt
1 jar spaghetti sauce
1 (6-oz.) can tomato paste
½ tsp. garlic salt
1 tsp. Italian seasoning
1 (3.5-oz.) pkg. pepperoni slices
3 cups mozzarella cheese

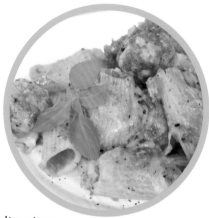

Cook pasta according to package directions (half the time if freezing). Set aside. In a skillet, combine browned ground beef, chopped onion, salt, spaghetti sauce, tomato paste, garlic salt, and Italian seasoning. Simmer 15 minutes. Combine pasta with meat sauce. Cut ¾ of the package of pepperoni into smaller pieces (4 triangles). Mix with pasta and meat sauce. Add 2 cups mozzarella. Pour mixture into a greased 9 × 13 pan. Top with remaining mozzarella and slices of pepperoni. If freezing, see directions below. Otherwise, cover and bake at 375 degrees for 30 minutes. Uncover and bake 10 minutes longer, or until bubbly.

Freezing directions: Cover with plastic wrap and then foil. Freeze. When baking, make sure to remove plastic wrap and then replace foil to bake.

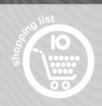

shopping list

- 10 (16-oz.) pkgs. spiral pasta
- 10 lbs. ground beef
- 10 onions
- Abt. ¼ cup salt
- 10 jars spaghetti sauce
- 10 (6-oz.) cans tomato paste
- 5 tsp. garlic salt
- Abt. ¼ cup Italian seasoning
- 10 (3.5-oz.) pkgs. pepperoni
- 7½ lbs. mozzarella cheese

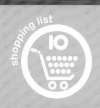

shopping list

- 30–40 lbs. rump roast

- 10 pkgs. Good Seasons Italian dressing mix

- 10 pkgs. au jus gravy mix

- Abt. ½ cup Italian seasoning

- 2½ Tbsp. pepper

Savory Italian Roast Beef Sandwiches

Fabulously flavorful!

3–4 lbs. rump roast
1 pkg. Good Seasons Italian Dressing Mix
1 cup water
1 pkg. au jus gravy mix
2 tsp. Italian seasoning
¼ tsp. pepper

Place roast in slow cooker. Mix together remaining ingredients and pour over roast. Cover and cook on low 4–6 hours or until soft enough to shred. If freezing, see directions below. Otherwise, shred and cook an additional hour. Serve on rolls or buns.

Freezing directions: Shred roast beef. Pour beef and juices in a gallon-size freezer bag and then freeze. Include hoagie buns with this meal.

Shredded Beef Burritos

Once prepared, these make quick and easy dinners or lunches!

2–3 lbs. beef roast
1 onion, chopped
1 (10-oz.) can chopped green chilies
2 (8-oz.) cans tomato sauce
1 Tbsp. chili powder
salt and pepper to taste
8 flour tortillas
refried beans
cheese

Place roast in slow cooker. Cook on low 8 hours until it will shred easily. (This is perfect to let slow cook all night.) Add remaining ingredients. Cook on low 2–3 hours. Spread meat filling on a tortilla. Add refried beans, grated cheese, and whatever toppings you prefer. If freezing, see directions below. Otherwise, wrap in foil and bake at 350 degrees for 10–15 minutes.

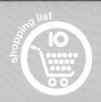

- Abt. 20–30 lbs. beef roast

- 10 onions

- 10 (10-oz.) cans chopped green chilies

- 20 (8-oz.) cans tomato sauce (160 oz.)

- Abt. ¾ cup chili powder

- 80 flour tortillas

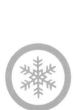

Freezing directions: Wrap each burrito in plastic wrap. Place several burritos in a gallon-size freezer bag. To prepare, remove individually and microwave for 2 minutes (still in plastic wrap). Or thaw, wrap in foil, and bake according to directions.

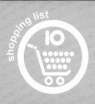

- 20 lbs. stew meat

- 20 cans French onion soup

- 20 cans cream of mushroom soup

- 10 pkgs. wide egg noodles

Steak and Noodles

This simple meal will impress the hubby and kids alike!

2 lbs. stew meat
2 cans French onion soup (undiluted)
2 cans cream of mushroom soup (undiluted)
1 pkg. wide egg noodles

Combine all ingredients in slow cooker, except noodles. Cook on low 6–8 hours. If freezing, see directions below. Serve over wide egg noodles.

Freezing directions: Let cool. Place in a gallon-size freezer bag and freeze. Include a package of wide egg noodles with this meal.

Stuffed Hard Rolls

These are a fun, unique way to have rolls with your dinner!

1 lb. ground beef, browned
1 can cream of mushroom soup
½ cup chopped onion
½ cup chopped celery
1 cup grated cheese
9 medium hard rolls

Stir together ground beef, mushroom soup, onion, celery, and cheese. If freezing, see directions below. Otherwise, carefully cut the rolls in half and hollow out the insides. Stir the inside pieces of rolls in with the meat mixture. Spoon meat mixture in one of the roll halves. Top with other half. Wrap in foil. Bake at 350 degrees for 15 minutes. Let sit 10 minutes before serving.

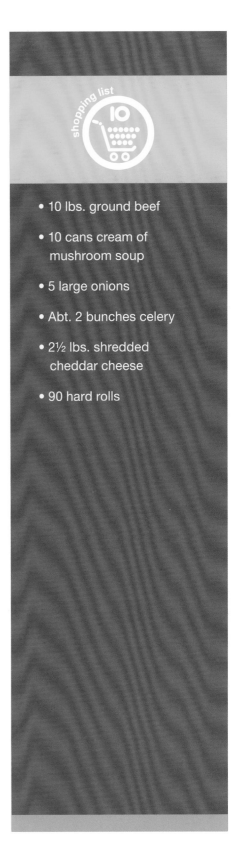

shopping list

- 10 lbs. ground beef

- 10 cans cream of mushroom soup

- 5 large onions

- Abt. 2 bunches celery

- 2½ lbs. shredded cheddar cheese

- 90 hard rolls

Freezing directions: Place meat mixture in a gallon-size freezer bag. Freeze. Include a package of hard rolls with this meal along with instructions on how to prepare.

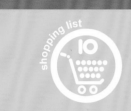
- 7½ cups brown sugar

- 10 (6-oz.) cans tomato paste

- 5 sweet onions

- 480 frozen meatballs

- 60 hoagie buns

- 2½ lbs. grated cheese

Sweet Onion Meatball Subs

This great flavor will be a hit!

1 cup water
¾ cup brown sugar
1 (6-oz.) can tomato paste
½ sweet onion, sliced
48 frozen meatballs
6 hoagie buns
1 cup grated cheese

Mix water, brown sugar, and tomato paste. Stir in onions and meatballs. If freezing, see directions below. Otherwise, cook in slow cooker on low 5–6 hours. Spoon meatballs with sauce onto toasted hoagie buns. Sprinkle with grated cheese.

Freezing Directions: Place in a gallon-size freezer bag and freeze. Include a bag of grated cheese and hoagie buns with this meal.

Taquitos for a Crowd

Make these for a crowd, or have them in the freezer
for a quick and easy meal or snack.

8–10 cups cooked, chopped roast beef (canned roast beef also works
    nicely)
2 cans black beans, drained and rinsed
2 cans corn, drained
4 cups shredded cheddar or Mexican blend cheese
3 cups salsa
60 flour tortillas
Abt. 32 oz. oil for frying

Slow cook roast 6–8 hours until it shreds and then chop finely. If you use a 6-pound rump roast, you should have plenty of meat. In a large bowl, mix beef, beans, corn, cheese, and salsa. In a frying pan, heat oil to medium heat. One at a time, using tongs, dip tortillas into hot oil for 5–10 seconds until it begins to bubble slightly. (You may have to use a spatula to get it out of the oil so it doesn't tear.) Set aside on paper towels. (Do only about 12 at a time; fill, roll, and repeat). Fill each tortilla with about ¼ cup of the mixture. (More or less if you want them thicker or thinner.) Roll tightly and place seam-side down on a cookie sheet. Makes about 60. If freezing, see directions below. Otherwise, bake at 400 degrees for 10–15 minutes.

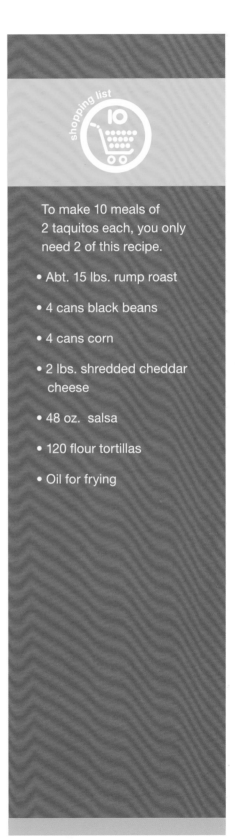

To make 10 meals of
2 taquitos each, you only
need 2 of this recipe.

• Abt. 15 lbs. rump roast

• 4 cans black beans

• 4 cans corn

• 2 lbs. shredded cheddar
  cheese

• 48 oz. salsa

• 120 flour tortillas

• Oil for frying

Freezing directions: When the cookie sheet is full, flash freeze. When firm, place in gallon-size freezer bags. To reheat, bake at 400 degrees for 20–25 minutes until heated through.

Chicken Recipes

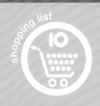
- 10 (12-oz.) pkgs. wide egg noodles

- 3 large onions

- 1¾ cups butter

- Abt. 15 lbs. boneless, skinless chicken breasts

- 20 cups frozen chopped broccoli

- 20 cans cream of chicken soup

- 5 cups milk

- 2½ tsp. dried thyme

- 5 tsp. salt

- Abt. ¼ cup pepper

- 5 lbs. shredded cheddar cheese

Broccoli Chicken Noodle Bake

Kid pleasing, Mom approved.

1 (12-oz.) pkg. wide egg noodles
¼ cup chopped onion
2 Tbsp. butter or margarine
2 cups cooked and cubed chicken breasts
2 cups frozen chopped broccoli
2 cans cream of chicken soup
½ cup milk
¼ tsp. dried thyme
½ tsp. salt
1 tsp. pepper
2 cups shredded cheddar cheese

Cook noodles according to package directions. (Half the time if freezing.) Drain. Sauté onion in butter. Add chicken, broccoli, soup, milk, and seasonings. Cook until broccoli is tender. Add noodles and mix well. If freezing, see directions below. Otherwise, place in a greased 9 × 13 pan. Cover and bake at 375 degrees for 30 minutes. Uncover, top with cheese, and bake an additional 10 minutes until cheese is melted.

Freezing directions: Place in a greased disposable aluminum pan. Cover and freeze. Include a bag of shredded cheese to top with.

Cheese Crisp Chicken

This chicken will be a family favorite for sure!

3 cups bread crumbs
½ cup grated cheddar cheese
½ cup shredded Parmesan cheese
1 tsp. salt
¼ tsp. pepper
6 boneless, skinless chicken breasts
½ cup melted butter

Topping:
¼ cup fresh shredded Parmesan cheese
2 Tbsp. melted butter

Mix together bread crumbs, cheeses, salt, and pepper. Dip chicken in melted butter and then in bread crumb mixture. Place in a 9 × 13 baking dish. Drizzle butter for topping over chicken and top with Parmesan cheese. If freezing, see directions below. Otherwise, bake at 350 degrees for 1 hour.

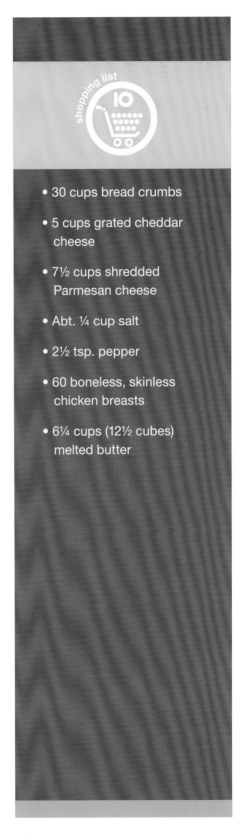

shopping list

- 30 cups bread crumbs
- 5 cups grated cheddar cheese
- 7½ cups shredded Parmesan cheese
- Abt. ¼ cup salt
- 2½ tsp. pepper
- 60 boneless, skinless chicken breasts
- 6¼ cups (12½ cubes) melted butter

Freezing directions: Place prepared chicken in a disposable pan, cover with foil, and freeze.

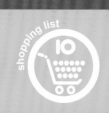

shopping list

- 2½ cups butter
- 5 large green peppers
- 10 small onions
- 10 cans cream of chicken soup
- 7½ cups milk
- Abt. 15 lbs. chicken
- 4 lbs. shredded cheddar cheese
- 10 pkgs. wide egg noodles

Chicken a La King

Fit for the kings, queens, princes, and princesses in your life!

¼ cup butter
½ cup diced green pepper
1 small onion, chopped
1 can cream of chicken soup
¾ cup milk
2 cups cooked chicken, cubed or shredded
1½ cups shredded cheese
noodles

In skillet, melt butter. Sauté green pepper and onion until tender. Stir in soup and milk. Blend well. Stir in chicken and cheese. Cook 5 minutes until heated through and cheese is melted. If freezing, see directions below. Otherwise, serve over noodles.

Freezing directions: Cool until warm. Place in gallon-size freezer bag and freeze. Include a package of noodles with this meal.

Chicken and Bean Burritos

Freeze these individually for a quick and yummy lunch.

4–6 boneless, skinless chicken breasts
1 pkg. taco seasoning
1 cup water
1 pkg. New Orleans style beans and
    rice mix
1 (30-count) pkg. flour tortillas
4 cups shredded cheddar cheese

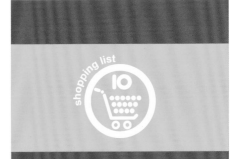

Place chicken and taco seasoning along with 1 cup of water in slow cooker. Cook until chicken shreds, about 4 hours. Shred and keep warm. Cook beans and rice mix according to package directions. Layer each tortilla with shredded chicken, beans, rice, and cheese. Roll up. If freezing, see directions below. Otherwise, microwave until cheese is melted and serve with salsa and sour cream, if desired.

Freezing directions: Wrap each burrito in plastic wrap. Place several in gallon-size freezer bags. To reheat, leave in plastic and heat in microwave for 2 minutes. This recipe will make enough for 3 family meals.

To make 10 meals of 8 burritos each, you only need 4 of this recipe.

- About 12 lbs. boneless, skinless chicken breasts

- 4 pkgs. taco seasoning

- 4 pkgs. New Orleans style beans and rice mix

- 120 flour tortillas

- 4 lbs. shredded cheddar cheese

- 5 large onions
- Abt. 2 cups butter
- Abt. 2¼ cups flour
- 4 qts. half and half
- Abt. 20 lbs. boneless, skinless chicken breasts
- Approx. 10 lbs. boneless ham
- 4 lbs. shredded cheddar cheese
- 5 cups dried bread crumbs
- 5 cups grated Swiss cheese

Chicken Cordon Bleu Casserole

This casserole is sure to please!

½ cup chopped onion
2 Tbsp. butter
3 Tbsp. flour
1½ cups (12-oz.) half and half
3 cups chicken, cooked and cubed
2 cups cubed ham
1½ cups shredded cheddar cheese

Topping:
½ cup dried bread crumbs
1 Tbsp. melted butter
½ cup grated Swiss cheese

Sauté onions in butter. Then add flour and mix until smooth. Stir in half and half and bring to a boil until thick, stirring constantly. In a separate bowl, mix together chicken, ham, and cheese. Pour sauce over and mix well. Mix together topping ingredients. If freezing, see directions below. Otherwise, pour into a 9 × 13 pan and sprinkle with topping. Bake at 350 degrees for 30 minutes.

Freezing directions: Place in a disposable pan and sprinkle with topping. Cover with foil and freeze.

Chicken Nuggets with a Kick

These have a slight kick, but nothing like you would expect!

¾ cup buttermilk (or just mix 1 Tbsp. lemon juice with regular milk)
⅓ cup hot sauce (like Tabasco)
1 tsp. seasoned salt
2 lbs. boneless, skinless chicken breasts cut into cubes
1 cup flour
¼ cup cornstarch
¼ cup corn flour
1 Tbsp. paprika
1 tsp. salt
1 tsp. pepper
¼ tsp. garlic powder
⅛ tsp. onion salt
oil (for frying)

In a gallon-size freezer bag, combine buttermilk, hot sauce, and seasoned salt. Add chicken cubes. Let refrigerate for 4 hours or overnight. In a large bowl, combine flour, cornstarch, corn flour, paprika, salt, pepper, garlic powder, and onion salt. Mix well. Dip chicken pieces in flour mixture until completely covered. Heat oil to 350 degrees and fry chicken pieces until golden brown. Drain on paper towel. If freezing, see directions below.

Freezing directions: Place all nuggets on a cookie sheet and place in freezer to flash freeze. When they are firm to the touch (about 2 hours), place in a gallon-size freezer bag and put back in freezer. To reheat, place on cookie sheet. Bake at 425 degrees for 15 minutes.

shopping list

- Abt. ½ gallon buttermilk
- 10 cups flour
- 2½ cups cornstarch
- 2½ cups corn flour
- Abt. ¾ cup paprika
- Abt. ¼ cup salt
- Abt. ¼ cup pepper
- 2½ tsp. garlic powder
- 1¼ tsp. onion salt
- oil
- 3 ⅓ cups hot sauce
- Abt. ¼ cup seasoned salt
- 20 lbs boneless, skinless chicken breasts

shopping list

- 10 cans cream of chicken soup
- 5 pints sour cream
- 10 cups milk
- 7½ cups mayonnaise
- Abt. 15 lbs. boneless, skinless chicken breasts
- 5 lbs. shredded cheddar cheese
- Abt. 2¼ cups parsley
- Abt. ¼ cup salt
- 5 tsp. pepper
- 1½ cups lemon juice
- 10 (16-oz.) pkgs. country pasta
- 7½ cups bread crumbs

Country Chicken Stroganoff Casserole

Creamy, cheesy, yummy!

1 can cream of chicken soup
1 cup sour cream
1 cup milk
¾ cup mayonnaise
2 cups cooked and cubed chicken
2 cups grated cheese
3 Tbsp. parsley
1 tsp. salt
½ tsp. pepper
2 Tbsp. lemon juice
16 oz. country pasta, cooked and drained
¾ cup bread crumbs

Combine all ingredients except bread crumbs. Pour into a 9 × 13 pan. Top with bread crumbs. If freezing, see directions below. Otherwise bake 45 minutes at 375 degrees.

Freezing directions: Undercook the pasta by about half the time required. Cover with foil and freeze.

Creamy Chicken and Rice Casserole

Potato chip crumbs make this casserole a hit!

1 cup chopped celery
1 onion, chopped
2 Tbsp. butter
1½ cups mayonnaise
1 can cream of chicken soup
½ cup milk
1 cup peas
1 Tbsp. lemon juice
1½ tsp. salt
sautéed veggies
3 cups cooked, cubed chicken
3 cups cooked rice
2 cups crushed potato chips

In a skillet, sauté celery and onion in butter until almost tender. In a bowl, combine mayonnaise, soup, milk, peas, lemon juice, and salt. Add sautéed veggies and mix well. Add chicken and cooked rice. Pour into a greased 9 × 13 pan. If freezing, see directions below. Otherwise, top with sprinkled potato chips and bake uncovered at 350 degrees for 30–40 minutes until bubbly.

Freezing directions: Do not place chips on casserole to freeze. Put them in a baggie and include them with the meal to top with before baking.

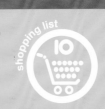

- Abt. 2 bunches celery
- 10 small onions
- Abt. 1½ cups butter
- 15 cups mayonnaise
- 10 cans cream of chicken soup
- 5 cups milk
- 10 cups peas
- Abt. ¼ cup lemon juice
- 5 Tbsp. salt
- Sautéed veggies
- Abt. 20 lbs. boneless, skinless chicken breasts
- 30 cups rice
- Abt. 5 bags potato chips

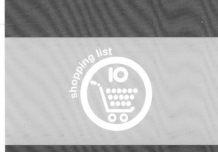
- 60 boneless, skinless chicken breasts

- 10 family-size cans cream of chicken soup

- 5 Bottles of Paul Newman's Lighten Up Honey Mustard dressing (or favorite dressing)

- 10 small bags baby carrots

- 10 pkgs. noodles

Crock-Pot Honey Mustard Chicken

You can substitute any of your favorite salad dressings in this recipe.

6 boneless, skinless chicken breasts
1 family-size can cream of chicken soup
½ bottle of your favorite honey mustard salad dressing (my favorite is Paul Newman's Lighten Up Honey Mustard dressing)
1 bag baby carrots

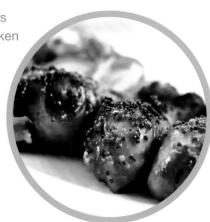

If freezing, see directions below.

Otherwise, put all ingredients together in slow cooker. Cook on low 6–8 hours. Break chicken into small pieces. Serve over noodles or rice.

Freezing directions: Place all ingredients in a gallon-size freezer bag and freeze. Include a package of noodles with this meal.

Fiesta Stuffed Chicken

This chicken has a delicious south-of-the-border taste!

6 boneless, skinless chicken breasts
1 (7-oz.) can chopped green chilies, drained
8 slices Monterey Jack cheese
1 cup bread crumbs
½ cup grated Parmesan cheese
2 Tbsp. chili powder
½ tsp. cumin
½ tsp. salt
¼ tsp. pepper
½ cup butter, melted

Pound each chicken breast to ¼-inch thickness. Sprinkle 2 teaspoons chopped green chilies and one slice of cheese on each chicken breast. Roll the chicken up tightly and secure with a toothpick. Combine remaining ingredients in a bowl, except butter. Dip each chicken roll in melted butter and then coat in bread crumb mixture. If freezing, see directions below. Otherwise, place seam-side down in a greased 9×13 pan and bake at 400 degrees for 30 minutes.

 Freezing directions: Place chicken seam-side down in a greased disposable pan. Cover with foil and freeze.

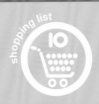

- 60 boneless, skinless chicken breasts

- 10 (7-oz.) cans chopped green chilies

- 80 slices (abt. 6 lbs.) Monterey Jack cheese

- 10 cups bread crumbs

- 5 cups grated Parmesan cheese

- Abt. 1½ cups chili powder

- 5 tsp. cumin

- 5 tsp. salt

- 2½ tsp. pepper

- 5 cups butter

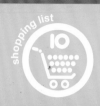
- 10 (32-oz.) pkgs. frozen shredded hash browns

- About ¼ cup salt

- 2½ tsp. pepper

- Abt. 20 lbs. chicken

- 5 pints sour cream

- 10 cans chicken broth

- 10 cans cream of chicken soup

- Abt. ½ cup bouillon granules

- 5 onions

- 5 red bell peppers

- Abt. ¼ cup garlic powder

Hash Brown Chicken Bake

This simple chicken and potato meal is filling on its own.

1 (32-oz.) pkg. frozen shredded hash browns
1 tsp. salt
¼ tsp. pepper
3 cups cooked, cubed chicken
1 cup sour cream
1 (15-oz.) can chicken broth
1 can cream of chicken soup
2 tsp. chicken bouillon granules
½ small onion, finely chopped
½ red bell pepper, finely chopped
1 tsp. garlic powder

Spread hash browns in a greased 9 × 13 pan. Sprinkle with salt and pepper. Place chicken cubes evenly over hash browns. In a medium-sized bowl, combine sour cream, chicken broth, cream of chicken soup, bouillon, onion, red pepper, and garlic powder. Pour over chicken and hash browns. If freezing, see directions below. Otherwise, bake at 350 degrees for 1 hour or until bubbly.

Freezing directions: Cover with foil and freeze.

Pork Recipes

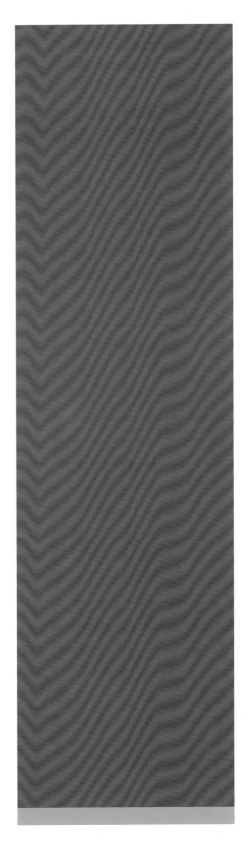

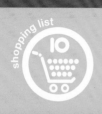

- 10 (16-oz.) pkgs. bow tie pasta
- Abt. 1½ cups butter
- Abt. 1½ cups flour
- 1 gallon + 1 quart milk
- 5 tsp. salt
- 2½ tsp. pepper
- 2½ tsp. nutmeg
- 10 lbs. shredded Monterey Jack or Cheddar cheese
- Abt. 10 lbs. boneless ham

Bow Tie Ham and Cheese

This is mac and cheese at its finest!

1 (16-oz.) pkg. bow tie pasta
2 Tbsp. butter
2 Tbsp. flour
2 cups milk
½ tsp. salt
¼ tsp. pepper
¼ tsp. ground nutmeg
4 cups shredded Monterey Jack or cheddar cheese
2 cups cubed ham

Cook pasta according to package directions (half the time if freezing). While pasta is cooking, melt butter in a saucepan over medium heat. Stir in flour until well blended. Add milk and stir constantly until thickened and bubbly. Remove from heat and stir in salt, pepper, nutmeg, and 3 cups of cheese. Add drained pasta and ham. Pour into a greased 9 × 13 pan. Sprinkle with remaining cheese. If freezing, see directions below. Otherwise, bake at 350 degrees for 30 minutes or until bubbly.

Freezing directions: Cover with foil and freeze.

Dad's Favorite Pork Chops

This is a meat and potatoes meal for the man in your life!

6 boneless pork chops
½ tsp. seasoned salt
½ tsp. garlic salt
2 Tbsp. olive oil
1 can cream of mushroom soup
½ cup sour cream
½ cup milk
½ tsp. pepper
1 (24-oz.) bag shredded hash browns
2 cups cheese
1 (2.8-oz.) can cheddar flavored French fried onions

Season pork chops with seasoned salt and garlic salt and then brown in olive oil. Meanwhile, in a large bowl, combine soup, milk, sour cream, and pepper. Stir in potatoes, 1 cup cheese, and half of the French fried onions. Place mixture in a greased 9 × 13 pan. Top potatoes with pork chops. If freezing, see directions below. Otherwise, bake covered for 40 minutes at 350 degrees. Uncover and sprinkle remaining cheese and onions over the pork chops. Bake for 5 more minutes.

Freezing directions: Place in a disposable pan, cover with foil, and freeze. Include remaining cheese and French fried onions with this meal.

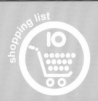

- 60 Boneless pork chops
- 5 tsp. seasoned salt
- 5 tsp. garlic salt
- Abt. 1½ cups olive oil
- 10 cans cream of mushroom soup
- 5 cups sour cream
- 5 cups milk
- 5 tsp. pepper
- 10 (24-oz.) bags shredded hash browns
- 5 lbs. shredded cheddar cheese
- 10 (2.8-oz.) cans Cheddar flavored French Fried onions

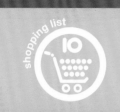

Shopping List 10

- 10 boxes of manicotti shells

- 10 small onions

- 1–2 bulbs or ¼ cup minced garlic

- 1¼ cups butter

- Abt. 15 lbs. boneless ham

- Abt. 2 lbs. butter

- 4½ cups flour

- Abt. 2 gallons milk

- 5 tsp. pepper

- 5 lbs. Swiss cheese

- 16 cups grated Parmesan cheese

Ham Stuffed Manicotti

One word: "Wow!"

14 manicotti shells
1 onion, chopped
2 cloves minced garlic
¼ cup butter
3 cups cubed ham
⅓ cup grated Parmesan cheese
6 Tbsp. butter
6 Tbsp. flour
3 cups milk
½ tsp. pepper
2 cups shredded Swiss cheese
½ cup grated Parmesan cheese

Cook manicotti according to package instructions (half the time if freezing). Drain and set aside. Sauté onion and garlic in butter. Add ham and cook for a few minutes. Set aside to cool slightly. Stir ⅓ cup Parmesan cheese into ham mixture. In a saucepan, melt 6 tablespoons butter. Stir in flour and heat until bubbly. Add milk and pepper. Whisk while cooking on medium to medium-high heat until thickened. Stir in Swiss cheese and remaining ½ cup Parmesan cheese. Mix a fourth of this cheese sauce with the ham mixture. Fill the manicotti shells with ham mixture. (A baby spoon works great for filling the shells without making a mess.) If freezing, see directions below. Otherwise, spread half of the remaining cheese sauce in the bottom of a greased 9 × 13 pan. Place filled shells in pan and cover with remaining sauce. Bake at 350 degrees for 30 minutes.

Freezing directions: Spread half of the remaining cheese sauce in the bottom of a greased disposable pan. Place filled shells in pan and cover with remaining sauce. Cover and freeze.

Hawaiian Pork

Aloha, taste buds!

3–4 lbs. boneless pork loin
1 tsp. nutmeg
½ tsp. paprika
½ cup ketchup
½ cup orange juice
4 Tbsp. honey
2 Tbsp. soy sauce
4 Tbsp. lemon juice
1½ Tbsp. cornstarch
¼ cup water

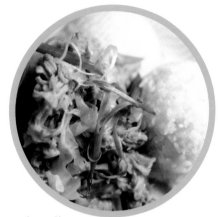

Place pork loin in slow cooker. Mix together all ingredients except cornstarch and water. Pour over roast. Cook on low 6–8 hours (or until able to shred). Shred pork. Pour juices in a saucepan. Heat to boil. Mix cornstarch with water and pour into sauce. Cook just until thickened. Mix with meat. If freezing, see directions below. Otherwise, serve over rice.

Freezing directions: Place in a gallon-size freezer bag and freeze.

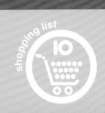

shopping list

- 30–40 lbs. pork loin
- Abt. ¼ cup nutmeg
- 5 tsp. paprika
- 5 cups ketchup
- 5 cups orange juice
- Abt. 3 cups honey
- Abt. 1½ cups soy sauce
- Abt. 3 cups lemon juice
- Abt. 1 cup cornstarch

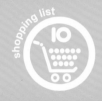
- 60 boneless pork chops

- 5 cups Honey Dijon mustard

- Abt. 1½ cups Worcestershire sauce

- 10 cups Italian bread crumbs

Honey Dijon Pork Chops

A different way to have your chops!

½ cup honey Dijon mustard
2 Tbsp. Worcestershire sauce
6 boneless pork chops
1 cup Italian bread crumbs

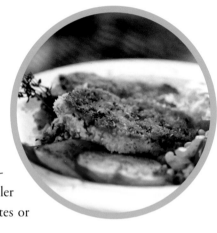

In a bowl, combine mustard and Worcestershire sauce. Dip each side of pork chop in mustard mixture and then in bread crumbs. If freezing, see directions below. Otherwise, place on broiler pan. Broil each side on low 10–15 minutes or until cooked through.

Freezing directions: Flash freeze these so they can be taken out and cooked individually, if desired. Place on a cookie sheet. Put in freezer until firm. Place in a gallon-size freezer bag and freeze.

Swedish Pork Roast

This is a delicious way to prepare a pork roast!

1 tsp. nutmeg
1 tsp. cinnamon
½ tsp. ginger
2 tsp. salt
1 clove garlic
½ cup brown sugar
½ cup apple cider vinegar
3–4 lbs. pork loin roast
2 onions, sliced
5 potatoes, peeled and sliced
4 carrots, sliced
4 bay leaves

Mix together the nutmeg, cinnamon, ginger, salt, garlic, brown sugar, and apple cider vinegar, creating spice mixture. If freezing, see directions below. Otherwise, place roast, onions, potatoes, carrots, and bay leaves in slow cooker, and pour spice mixture over the top. Cook on low in slow cooker for 6–8 hours. Remove bay leaves. Make gravy with drippings.

Freezing directions: Place roast, onions, potatoes, carrots, and bay leaves in a gallon-size freezer bag. Pour spice mixture over the roast. Freeze.

- Abt. ¼ cup nutmeg

- Abt. ¼ cup cinnamon

- 5 tsp. ginger

- Abt. ½ cup salt

- 10 cloves or 5 tsp. minced garlic

- 5 cups brown sugar

- 5 cups apple cider vinegar

- 10 3–4 lbs. pork roasts

- 20 onions

- 50 potatoes

- 40 carrots

- 40 bay leaves

- 60 boneless pork chops

- 10 pkgs. taco seasoning

- 2¼ cups vegetable oil

- 10 jars apricot jam

- 10 cups salsa

- 10 pkgs. tortillas

Sweet and Spicy Pork Tenders

These tender pork pieces are a hit with the kids and easy on Mom!

6 boneless pork chops
1 pkg. taco seasoning
3 Tbsp. oil
1 jar apricot jam
1 cup salsa

Cut pork into bite-sized pieces. Place pork and taco seasoning in a plastic bag and shake well. Brown meat in oil. Add apricot jam and salsa and simmer for 15 minutes. If freezing, see directions below. Otherwise, serve over steamed rice.

 Freezing directions: Place in a gallon-size bag and freeze. Include a package of tortillas.

Sweet Crock-Pot Pork Chops

These pork chops are tender and "sa-weet"!

8 boneless pork loin chops
½ cup brown sugar
½ cup chopped sweet onion
½ cup ketchup
½ cup barbecue sauce
½ cup French salad dressing
½ cup honey
rice

If freezing, see directions below. Otherwise, place pork chops in slow cooker. Combine the remaining ingredients and pour over pork chops. Cook on low 6–8 hours. Serve over rice.

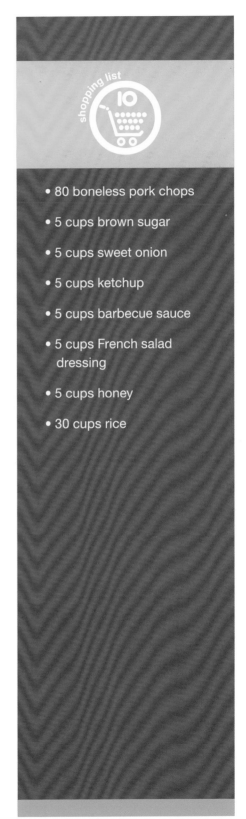

shopping list

- 80 boneless pork chops

- 5 cups brown sugar

- 5 cups sweet onion

- 5 cups ketchup

- 5 cups barbecue sauce

- 5 cups French salad dressing

- 5 cups honey

- 30 cups rice

Freezing directions: Place pork chops in a gallon-size freezer bag. Combine remaining ingredients and pour over pork chops. Freeze. Include 3 cups rice with this meal.

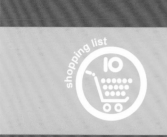
- 30–40 pork loins

- 20 cups (160 oz.) salsa

- 20 cups brown sugar

- 14 (12-oz.) cans Dr. Pepper

Sweet Pork Burritos

This recipe also makes fabulous salads!

3–4 lbs. pork loin roast
2 cups salsa
2 cups brown sugar
2 cups Dr. Pepper

Place pork loin in slow cooker. Mix together salsa, brown sugar, and Dr. Pepper. Pour 4 cups of mixture over pork. Cook on low all day. About 1 hour before serving, shred pork and add remaining mixture. Cook for 1 more hour. If freezing, see directions below. Otherwise, serve on tortillas with black beans and whatever toppings your family likes.

Freezing directions: Place in gallon-size freezer bag and freeze.

Soup Recipes

shopping list

- 10 lbs. ground beef
- 5 cups dried bread crumbs
- 5 cups Parmesan cheese
- 10 onions
- 20 cloves or 10 tsp. minced garlic
- Abt. ¾ cup dried parsley
- Abt. ½ cup dried basil
- 5 tsp. salt
- 10 eggs
- Abt. 1½ cups olive oil
- 10 ribs celery
- 9 (48-oz.) cartons chicken broth
- 3 (28-oz.) cans crushed tomatoes
- Abt. ¼ cup Italian seasoning
- 5 tsp. salt
- 5 cups alphabet pasta

ABC Meatball Soup

Learn while you eat!

Meatballs:
1 lb. ground beef
½ cup dried bread crumbs
½ cup Parmesan cheese
2 Tbsp. chopped onion
1 clove minced garlic
1 Tbsp. dried parsley
2 tsp. dried basil
½ tsp. salt
1 large egg, beaten

Combine all meatball ingredients and mix well. Shape into balls. Place on a cookie sheet and bake at 350 degrees for 25 minutes.

Soup:
2 Tbsp. olive oil
1 small onion, chopped
1 rib celery, chopped
1 clove garlic, minced
5 cups chicken broth
1 cup crushed tomatoes
1 tsp. Italian seasoning
½ tsp. salt
½ cup alphabet pasta

Heat olive oil in a large saucepan. Add onion, celery, and garlic. Cook over medium heat for 8–10 minutes. Add remaining ingredients except for pasta. Add meatballs. If freezing, see directions below. Otherwise, bring to a simmer. Add pasta and cook for 8–10 minutes.

Freezing directions: Pour into a gallon-size freezer bag and freeze. Include a bag of the alphabet pasta with this meal to be added when cooking.

Autumn Soup

This is the perfect hearty meal for a cool autumn day.

1 lb. ground beef
1 small onion
1 cup carrots, sliced
3 stalks celery, sliced
1 cup canned or frozen corn
4 potatoes, diced
1 quart stewed and diced tomatoes
1 can tomato sauce
1 Tbsp. oregano
1 Tbsp. basil

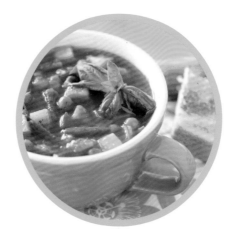

Brown ground beef with onion. Drain. If freezing, see directions below. Otherwise, add all ingredients to slow cooker and cook 4 hours or until potatoes and carrots are tender. Add salt and pepper to taste.

 Freezing directions: Place all ingredients in a gallon-size freezer bag and freeze. Instead of adding potatoes to this recipe, consider including frozen cubed hash browns that can be added when cooking. Otherwise, the potatoes get a little mushy.

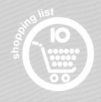

shopping list

- 10 lbs. ground beef
- 10 onions
- Abt. 15 carrots
- Abt. 3 bunches celery
- 10 cups corn
- 40 potatoes
- 10 quarts stewed and diced tomatoes
- 10 (8-oz.) cans tomato sauce
- Abt. ¾ cups oregano
- Abt. ¾ cups basil

- 10 onions

- 1¼ cups butter

- 30 (14-oz.) cans chicken broth

- 20 cans cream of chicken soup

- 10 (12-oz.) cans evaporated milk

- 10 lbs. Velveeta cheese cut in cubes

- 10 (24-oz.) bags frozen shredded hash browns

- 40 oz. pre-cooked bacon bits

Cheesy Potato Soup

Super easy and super cheesy!

1 onion, finely chopped
2 Tbsp. butter
3 (14-oz.) cans chicken broth
2 cans cream of chicken soup
1 (12-oz.) can evaporated milk
1 lb. Velveeta cheese, cut into cubes
1 bag frozen cubed hash browns
1 (4-oz.) pkg. pre-cooked bacon bits (not imitation)

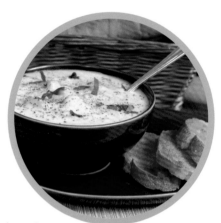

Sauté onion in butter. Add chicken broth and bring to a boil. Add soup and evaporated milk and bring to a boil. Add cheese and heat until melted. Add hash browns and bacon bits. If freezing, see directions below. Otherwise, simmer until potatoes are cooked through.

 Freezing directions: Place in a gallon-size freezer bag and freeze.

Hungry Hamburger Soup

This is hearty and flavorful, perfect for even the hungriest.

1 lb. ground beef, browned
3 cups water
1 cup chopped celery
1 cup shoestring carrots
1 can tomato sauce
1 Tbsp. soy sauce
1 pkg. dry onion soup mix
¼ tsp. pepper
¼ tsp. oregano
¼ tsp. basil
¼ tsp. seasoned salt
½ cup small shell pasta (cooked according to package instructions)

If freezing, see directions below. Otherwise, mix all ingredients together in a large saucepan except noodles. Simmer until vegetables are tender. Add cooked noodles. Cook another 10 minutes.

 Freezing directions: Place all ingredients except pasta in a gallon-size freezer bag and freeze. Include uncooked pasta with this meal. Include instructions to simmer until veggies are tender, and then add cooked pasta.

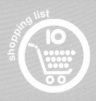

shopping list

- 10 lbs. ground beef
- Abt. 2 bunches celery
- 10 cups shoestring carrots
- 10 (8-oz.) cans tomato sauce
- Abt. ¾ cup soy sauce
- 10 pkgs. dry onion soup mix
- 2½ tsp. pepper
- 2½ tsp. oregano
- 2½ tsp. basil
- 2½ tsp. seasoned salt
- 5 cups small shell pasta

- 30 boneless, skinless chicken breasts

- Abt. ¼ cup minced garlic

- 10 onions

- 20 (16-oz.) cans chicken broth

- 10 (16-oz.) jars salsa

- 5 cups instant rice

- Abt. ¼ cup oregano

- Abt. ¼ cup salt

- 10 cans corn

- 10 cans black beans

- 10 (4-oz.) cans green chilies

- 10 pints sour cream

- 10 limes

Sour Cream and Lime Chicken Soup

The lime adds the perfect touch!

3 chicken breasts
2 cloves garlic
1 onion, chopped
1 cup water
32 oz. chicken broth
16 oz. salsa
½ cup instant rice
1 tsp. oregano
1 tsp. salt
1 can corn
1 can black beans
1 (4-oz.) can green chilies
juice from 1 lime
1 (16-oz.) tub sour cream

Cook chicken, garlic, and onion with olive oil. Add cooked chicken to a pot with water and chicken broth. Bring to a boil. Add salsa, instant rice, oregano, and salt. Simmer for 5 minutes. Add corn, black beans, and green chilies. If freezing, see directions below. Otherwise, squeeze the juice from the lime into the tub of sour cream. Drop a tablespoon or more of sour cream on top of each bowl when serving.

Freezing directions: Let soup cool. Pour into a gallon-size freezer bag and freeze. Include the tub of sour cream and a fresh lime with this meal.

Tex-Mex Chili

Super easy and hearty for cold winter days.

1 lb. ground beef, browned
1 finely chopped onion
1 clove minced garlic
1 (15-oz.) can tomato sauce
1 cup salsa
1½ Tbsp. chili powder
1 Tbsp. cider vinegar
1 Tbsp. brown sugar
2 tsp. Worcestershire sauce
¼ tsp. pepper
2 cans kidney beans, rinsed
2 cups frozen whole kernel corn

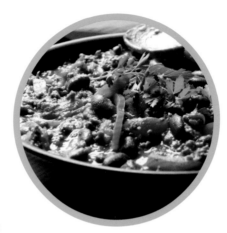

Mix all ingredients together in slow cooker. If freezing, see directions below. Otherwise, cook 6–8 hours on low. Serve topped with grated cheese.

 Freezing directions: Place all ingredients in a gallon-size freezer bag and freeze.

shopping list

- 10 lbs. ground beef
- 10 onions
- 5 tsp. minced garlic
- 10 (15-oz.) cans tomato sauce
- 10 cups salsa (80 oz.)
- Abt. 1 cup chili powder
- Abt. ¾ cup cider vinegar
- Abt. ¾ cup brown sugar
- About ½ cup Worcestershire sauce
- 2½ tsp. pepper
- 20 cans kidney beans
- 20 cups frozen corn

shopping list

- 15 to 20 lbs. turkey or chicken
- 10 onions
- 5 tsp. minced or 10 cloves garlic
- 20 carrots
- Abt. 2 bunches celery
- 20 potatoes (or 2 pkgs. frozen cubed hash browns)
- Abt. 26 oz. tomato sauce
- 10 cans creamed corn
- 10 cans whole kernel corn
- 20 (16-oz.) cans chicken broth
- 1½ cups dried parsley
- Abt. ¼ cup salt

Turkey Corn Chowder

You can also use chicken in this comfort food recipe.

2–3 cups cooked and cubed chicken or turkey
(or canned chicken or turkey)
1 onion, chopped
1 clove garlic, minced
2 carrots, sliced (or use carrot matchsticks)
2 ribs celery, chopped
2 medium potatoes, cubed (if freezing,
don't add these until ready to cook)
⅓ cup tomato sauce
1 can creamed corn
1 can whole kernel corn, drained
4 cups chicken broth
2 Tbsp. dried parsley
1 tsp. salt

Combine all ingredients. If freezing, see directions below. Otherwise, simmer on stove for 30 minutes or until vegetables are tender.

Freezing directions: Combine all ingredients except potatoes. Place in a gallon-size freezer bag and freeze. Replace the potatoes with half the package of frozen cubed hash browns.

White Chili with Chicken

A great twist on chili, perfect for a chilly night!

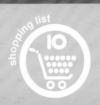

4 boneless, skinless chicken breasts
2 cans corn
2 cans northern white beans, drained and rinsed
1 small can green chilies
3 cups water
3 chicken-flavored bouillon cubes
1 medium onion, chopped
1 tsp. minced garlic
1 tsp. basil
1 tsp. oregano
1 tsp. cumin
1 tsp. salt
2 Tbsp. butter
juice from 1 lime
2 Tbsp. fresh cilantro
½ cup sour cream

Place all ingredients except lime juice, cilantro, and sour cream in a slow cooker. Cook 6–8 hours on low until chicken will shred. Shred chicken. Add lime juice and cilantro. Cook one more hour. Just before serving, add sour cream. If freezing, see directions below. This will make enough for 2 families.

Freezing directions: Cool. Place in gallon-size freezer bags, and freeze.

shopping list

- Abt. 20 lbs. boneless, skinless chicken breasts

- 10 cans corn

- 10 cans northern white beans

- 5 (4-oz.) cans diced green chilies

- 15 chicken flavored bouillon cubes

- 5 onions

- Abt. 5 tsp. minced garlic

- Abt. 5 tsp. basil

- Abt. 5 tsp. oregano

- Abt. 5 tsp. cumin

- Abt. 5 tsp. salt

- ⅔ cups butter

- 5 limes

- 1 bunch cilantro

- 2½ cups sour cream

Additional Recipes

Breads

These are recipes that are usually passed down through generations.
Everyone remembers Grandma's rolls or bread.

Shape these into dinner rolls and flash freeze. When frozen, place several in freezer bag and use as many as you need at a future time. Thaw and bake according to directions!

30-minute rolls

You can literally have homemade rolls on the table in 30 minutes, and you can even save half the dough for cinnamon rolls for dessert. Use it for all your dough needs, including pizza crust and breadsticks.

3½ cups warm water
1 cup oil
6 Tbsp. yeast
¾ cup sugar or honey
1½ tsp. salt
3 eggs
10½ cups flour

Mix together water, oil, yeast, and sugar (or honey), and let rest for 10 minutes. Add salt and eggs. Gradually add flour. Shape into dinner rolls. Place on pan and let rest for 10 minutes. Bake at 400 degrees for 10 minutes. Brush with melted butter. Makes about 60 rolls.

Jump for Joy Cornbread

This recipe has been known to make children jump for joy!

1 cup milk
2 eggs, beaten
½ cup butter, melted
½ cup cornmeal
½ tsp. baking powder
2 cups biscuit mix (like Bisquick)
½ cup sugar

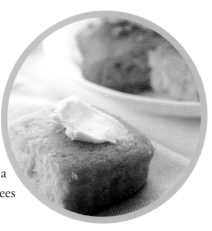

Combine all ingredients. Spread into a greased 8 × 8 pan and bake at 350 degrees for 30 minutes or until golden brown.

Great with chili on a cold day, or any day you want your children to jump for joy!

Make a double batch to freeze some for later!

Pumpkin Cranberry Bread

This bread screams, "Fall is here!" I start craving this about mid-October, and the craving lasts until the new year! Hmmm . . . maybe that explains why I have the same New Year's resolution every year!

4 eggs
½ cup vegetable oil
3 cups sugar
1 (16-oz.) can pumpkin
3¾ cups flour
2 tsp. baking soda
1 tsp. salt
1⅓ Tbsp. pumpkin pie spice
2 cups whole fresh cranberries (or substitute chocolate chips)
1 cup chopped nuts, optional

In a large bowl, beat eggs. Add oil and mix well. Blend in sugar and pumpkin. In a separate bowl, sift together dry ingredients. Add to pumpkin mixture. Fold in cranberries and nuts. Pour into 2 greased loaf pans. Bake at 350 degrees for 75 minutes or until toothpick inserted in center comes out clean. Cool 5 minutes and remove from pans to continue cooling.

Salads

A great way to get kids to eat broccoli is to tell them that the broccoli pieces are little trees. Have your kids eat off the leaves.

Broccoli Salad

Many people make a special dessert or salad for big family gatherings or potlucks. Sometimes I skip the meat and just go for the salads, so I have room to try them all! This one makes everyone say, "I've got to get that recipe!"

1 cup slivered almonds
1 Tbsp. butter
4–5 cups broccoli, cut into small pieces
2 large Granny Smith apples sliced and chopped
½ cup chopped green onions
1 cup craisins

Dressing:
1½ cups mayonnaise
⅔ cup sugar
1 tsp. salt
2 Tbsp. cider vinegar

Fry almonds in butter until golden brown. Mix remaining salad ingredients together. In separate bowl, mix together dressing ingredients and then pour over salad.

Snicker Salad

This is another favorite because if you call chocolate a salad, it makes it healthy, right?

5 apples, cut in bite-size pieces
3 Snicker bars, cut in bite-size pieces
1 small tub of Cool Whip

Mix all ingredients together and serve.

Get creative and add your own touches to this salad!

This salad is perfect for any meal. Use the dressing on any green salad.

Swiss Tossed Salad

Everyone wants the recipe for this salad!

Salad:
1 bunch romaine lettuce, torn
½ cup sliced almonds
1 cup grated Swiss cheese

Dressing:
⅓ cup white vinegar
¾ cup sugar
2 Tbsp. prepared mustard
1 tsp. grated onion
dash of salt
1 cup oil
1 tsp. poppy seeds

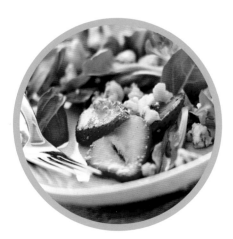

Mix together salad ingredients. In a blender, combine vinegar, sugar, mustard, onion, and salt. Cover and process until well blended. While processing, gradually add oil in a steady stream. Stir in poppy seeds. Serve over salad.

Party Recipes

This is even better the next day! (If there is any left.)

Caramel Corn

Family parties, game nights, movie nights, or get-togethers are always great memory makers. Keep the ingredients on hand to make this yummy, gooey caramel corn anytime you have an excuse.

2 cups brown sugar
1 cup light corn syrup
dash of salt
½ cup butter
1 can sweetened condensed milk
large bowl of popcorn (about 1 cup kernels before popped)

Boil brown sugar, corn syrup, salt, and butter together for 5–6 minutes on medium to medium-high heat. Remove from heat and stir in sweetened condensed milk. Pour over a large bowl of popped popcorn and mix well.

Alfredo Fondue

Bring this to game nights, and it will be the first to go!

1½ cups milk
2 (8-oz.) pkgs. cream cheese
½ tsp. garlic salt
½ tsp. salt
¾ cup grated Parmesan cheese

Blend the milk and cream cheese together. Heat slowly. Add salt and garlic salt. When bubbly, add Parmesan. Keep warm and serve with torn French bread, pretzels, crackers, broccoli, or whatever your heart desires!

If you eat this at a party, it has no calories!

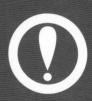

You'll be the hit of the party!

Seven-Layer Dip

This popular dip is always a favorite.

1st layer: 1 large can of refried beans mixed with 1 cup salsa
2nd layer: 2 cups guacamole
3rd layer: 2 cups sour cream mixed with ½ cup mayo
　　　　　　and 1 pkg. taco seasoning
4th layer: 3 cups grated cheddar cheese
5th layer: diced tomatoes
6th layer: sliced black olives
7th layer: chopped green onions

Spread layer 1 in a 9 × 13 pan, followed by layers 2 and then 3. Top with remaining layers in order. Chill for 1–4 hours. Serve with tortilla chips.

Party Casserole

Why is a casserole in with party recipes? Well, the definition of casserole is many yummy things mixed together to make something yummier!

1 large bag peanut M&Ms
1 bag pretzels
1 can party peanuts
1 bag Bugles

Add anything else your heart desires! You could get creative with this and add popcorn, Reese's Pieces, Twizzler Bites, or Dots—anything bite-sized that is sweet, salty, or chocolaty. This will be devoured when set in the middle of any table at game night!

Get creative with this. You could put it in clear party cups to look cute.

This stays fresh in the fridge for several days, and it even freezes well. Great for a healthy snack!

Corn Salsa (Cowboy Caviar)

So good, you can eat it with or without the chips!

2 cans corn, drained
2 cans black beans, rinsed
1 red bell pepper, chopped
1 green bell pepper, chopped
1 small onion, chopped
½ bottle Hendrickson's dressing (original sweet vinegar and olive oil)

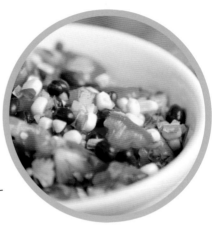

Mix all together and chill. Serve with tortilla chips.

Special Occasion Recipes

Every family has special occasion recipes. Whether it's your child's favorite on his birthday, a barbecue for Father's Day or Super Bowl Sunday, or a traditional family dish for Christmas dinner, it's just not the same without that special recipe.

These beans are always paired with Dad's Potato Salad.

Dad's Super Bowl Baked Beans

4 (15-oz.) cans pork and beans
1½ cups ketchup
2 cups brown sugar
2 tsp. dry mustard
Polish sausage or Little Smokies, cut in pieces

Mix all ingredients together and bake at 350 degrees for 1 hour, or slow cook on low for 3 hours.

Dad's Super Bowl Potato Salad

8 cups cubed potatoes, boiled and cooled
8 hard boiled eggs, diced
2 cups Miracle Whip
2 Tbsp. horseradish mustard

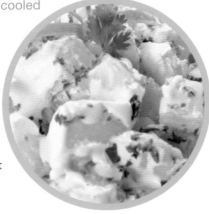

Place cooled potatoes and eggs in a medium-size bowl. Mix together Miracle Whip and horseradish mustard. Mix into potatoes and eggs. Chill 1 hour for best flavor.

This kid-friendly potato salad will please anyone.

I always double this and freeze one lasagna.

Birthday Dinner Lasagna

If you ask me what my favorite meal that my mom makes, this is it!
I haven't found a lasagna that even comes close!

Sauce:
1½ lb. ground beef, browned
1 tsp. parsley
1 tsp. salt
2 (6-oz.) cans tomato paste
1 clove minced garlic
1 tsp. basil
1 (1 lb.) can stewed tomatoes or 4
    small cans tomato sauce

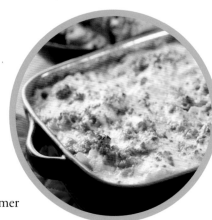

Mix together sauce ingredients and simmer until thick.

Cheese Mix:
3 cups cottage cheese
2 tsp. parsley
1 tsp. salt
2 beaten eggs
1 cup Parmesan cheese
½ tsp. pepper
1 lb. shredded mozzarella cheese

Combine cheese mix ingredients together, except the mozzarella.

Boil approximately 8 lasagna noodles. Cover bottom of a greased 9 × 13 pan with 4 noodles. Cover noodles with half of cheese mixture, half of mozzarella cheese, and half of meat sauce. Repeat layers. Bake at 375 degrees for 45 minutes. Let sit 15 minutes before serving.

Swedish Kringle

Christmas isn't the same without Swedish Kringle!

Part 1:
1 cup flour
2 Tbsp. water
½ cup butter or margarine

Mix ingredients together. Divide in half. With your fingers, shape into a flat and thin oval shapes. These should both fit on a big cookie sheet.

Part 2:
1 cup water
½ cup butter
1 cup flour
3 eggs
½ tsp. lemon extract

In a medium saucepan, bring water and butter to boil and remove from heat. Add flour and mix until smooth. Add eggs, one at a time. Add lemon extract. Spread over part one. Bake at 350 degrees for minutes. Don't overcook, so watch until golden brown and remove from oven.

Frosting:
1 cup powdered sugar
1 Tbsp. butter, softened
2 Tbsp. evaporated milk
½ tsp. lemon extract
food coloring (optional)

Mix frosting ingredients together and drizzle over warm pastry. Top with slivered almonds.

This is great all year, but especially at Christmastime!

You could half this recipe for a 9 x 9 pan.

Berry Buckle

This breakfast cake is fantastic! Whoever invented the idea that cakes and pastries were for breakfast is my hero!

1½ cups sugar
½ cup shortening
2 eggs
1 cup milk
4 tsp. baking powder
1 tsp. salt
4 cups flour
4 cups frozen mixed berries, thawed

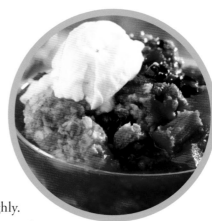

Mix sugar, shortening, and eggs thoroughly. Stir in milk. In separate bowl, mix dry ingredients and add to mixture. Gently fold in berries. Pour into a greased and floured 9 × 13 pan.

Topping:
⅔ cup flour
1 cup sugar
1 tsp. cinnamon
butter

Mix together flour, sugar, and cinnamon, and sprinkle over batter. Dot generously with butter. Bake at 375 degrees for 50–60 minutes.

Desserts

These are usually the recipes that are requested at birthdays and family nights. Desserts always bring people together, talking and laughing!

Frozen Raspberry Dessert (The $5 Dessert)

¾ cup brown sugar
1 cup toasted coconut
½ cup melted butter
4 cups crisped rice cereal
½ gallon vanilla ice cream,
  softened

Mix brown sugar, coconut, butter, and cereal together. Spread half of the mixture on the bottom of a 9 × 13 pan. Press softened ice cream onto cereal mixture. Top with the remaining cereal mixture. Cover and freeze.

Raspberry topping:
2 pkgs. frozen raspberries, thawed
water
1 cup sugar
4 tsp. lemon juice
4 Tbsp. cornstarch

Thaw raspberries and save juice. Use juice and enough water to make 1 cup. Bring to a boil, and add sugar and lemon juice. Mix cornstarch with a little water and slowly pour into boiling sauce. Cook until thick. Cool and serve over each piece of ice cream dessert.

Lemon Bars

A tip for eating lemon bars: do not inhale as you put it in your mouth! You'll know why!

2 cups flour
½ cup powdered sugar
1 cup butter
4 eggs
2 cups sugar
⅓ cup lemon juice
½ cup flour
½ tsp. baking powder

Blend together 2 cups flour, powdered sugar, and butter. Press into a 9 × 13 pan and bake at 350 degrees for 20 minutes, or until golden brown. Beat together eggs, sugar, and lemon juice. Add flour and baking powder. Pour over baked crust and then return to oven and bake 20–25 minutes. Sprinkle with powdered sugar.

These are great to make for potlucks because you always have the ingredients on hand.

They'll never know these are from a mix!

Easy Mint Brownies

Every Christmastime I start craving these and make them constantly during the holiday. They make a lot, so you can get several plates out of them for neighbor treats!

2 pkgs. chocolate fudge cake mix
1 cup butter, melted
2 eggs

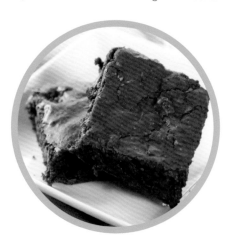

Mix together. Press in an 11 × 17 cookie sheet. Bake at 350 degrees for 10–12 minutes. Don't overbake.

Frosting:
1 tub white frosting
1 tsp. peppermint extract
green food coloring

Mix together. Frost cooled brownies.

Topping:
1 cup milk chocolate chips
4 Tbsp. butter
2 Tbsp. milk

Melt together in microwave. Drizzle over frosted brownies. Cool until chocolate is set.

Summer Slush

This slush recipe will have you dreaming of a hot summer day on the beach.

4 cups sugar
6 cups water
5 mashed bananas
1 quart pineapple juice
1 can frozen lemonade
1 can frozen orange juice
lemon-lime soda

Boil together sugar and water. Add remaining ingredients except soda and freeze until slushy. Spoon into cups and pour soda over the top.

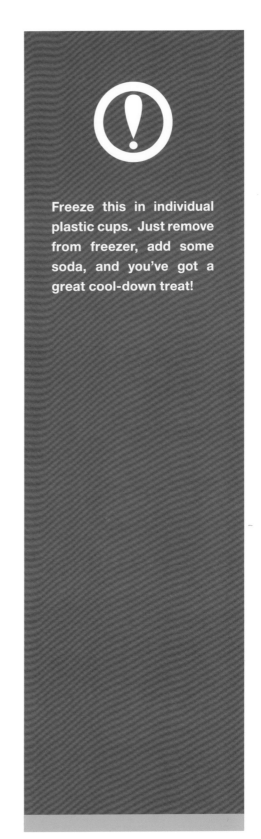

Freeze this in individual plastic cups. Just remove from freezer, add some soda, and you've got a great cool-down treat!

Index

*Italics indicate slow cooker recipes

About the Author

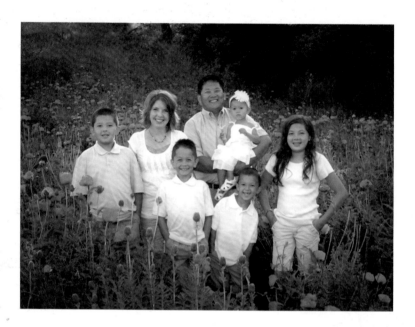

Suzie Roberts is one of those busy mothers who knows how challenging (not to mention boring!) putting dinner on the table night after night can be. She started her own Make-Ahead Meal Group in 2004 and became such a believer in this method of cooking that she decided to share her success with others. She continues to come up with creative and fun ways to give her more time to spend with family and friends. Suzie lives in Perry, Utah, with her husband, David, and their five children, Kyra, Kuen, Tatem, Bryson, and Mylee.